The National Council Licensure Examination For Practical Nurses

The National Council Licensure Examination For Practical Nurses

Prepared by the National Council of
State Boards of Nursing

Patricia Ann Winberg, R.N., B.S.N.
Nancy J. Miller, R.N., M.S.

with review of questions and rationale
for the third edition by

Karen W. Beaver, Ed.D, R.N.- C.
Helen L. Kelley, L.P.N.
Patricia Maggard, L.P.N.
Jacqueline Mitchell, R.N., B.S.N., M.Ed.

CHICAGO REVIEW PRESS

Library of Congress Cataloging-in-Publication Data

Winberg, Patricia Ann.
    National Council licensure examination for practical nurses / prepared by
National Council of State Boards of Nursing ; Patricia Ann Winberg, Nancy J.
Miller ; with review of questions and rationale for the third edition by Karen W.
Beaver . . . [et al]. — 3rd ed.
        p. cm.
    Rev. ed. of: National Council licensure examination for practical nurses / pre-
pared by the National Council of State Boards of Nursing; Eileen McQuaid
Dvorak, Ray E. Showalter. 2nd ed. c 1985.
    ISBN 1-55652-094-8: $9.95
    1. Practical nursing—Examinations, questions, etc. 2. National Council of State
Boards of Nursing (U.S.)—Examinations—Study guides.   I. Miller, Nancy J.,
R.N.   II. Beaver, Karen W.   III. Dvorak, Eileen McQuaid. National Council
licensure examination for practical nurses.   IV. National Council of State
Boards of Nursing (U.S.)   V. Title.
    [DNLM: 1. Licensure, Nursing—United States—examination questions. 2.
Nursing, Practical—examination questions.]
RT62.D86 1990
610.73'069'3076—dc20
DNLM/DLC
for Library of Congress   90-2379
                                                                   CIP

Contents

Acknowledgments

The authors wish to recognize all the former authors, contributors, reviewers, and licensure candidates who devoted time and energy to help make this book achieve the goal of helping new candidates for licensure as practical/vocational nurses to understand licensure examination development.

To the many who have added to the content of this book throughout its former and present editions, we affirm that the quality would not have been maintained without you.

The ongoing support of the National Council Board of Directors and the active involvement of selected National Council staff over the years have continued unabated. To all of you, we say thank you.

Nancy J. Miller, R.N., M.S.
Assistant Director of Testing Services

Introduction

This book is designed to provide you, a candidate for practical/vocational nurse licensure, with as much information as possible about the examination you must take as part of the process of becoming licensed to practice nursing in the United States.

The examination is the National Council Licensure Examination for Practical Nurses, more briefly known as NCLEX-PN. It is administered by boards of nursing in each of the United States and the U.S. territories of Guam, the Virgin Islands, American Samoa, and Commonwealth of Northern Mariana Islands, all of which will be referred to in this book as states for the purpose of simplicity.

The organization responsible for preparing NCLEX-PN and its counterpart for licensed registered nurses—the National Council Licensure Examination for Registered Nurses (NCLEX-RN)—is the National Council of State Boards of Nursing, Inc. Founded in 1978, the National Council consists of sixty-one Member Boards of Nursing, each of whom has been given responsibility by their state legislatures to regulate nursing practice in their own states. That responsibility includes not only regulating the practice of nurses already licensed but also determining who may enter into the practice of nursing.

Entry into the practice of nursing, as with any licensed profession, is regulated by states for the purpose of protecting the public from those who are unable to practice nursing safely and effectively. Therefore, candidates for licensure are asked by boards of nursing to provide evidence of their ability to deliver effective nursing care.

The primary evidence requires, along with a degree or diploma from a board-approved nursing education program, the successful completion of NCLEX-PN, which has been developed by the National Council under the direction of its Member Boards to test a licensure candidate's capabilities for

A General Description of the NCLEX-PN

National Council of State Boards of Nursing

NCLEX-PN

safe and effective entry-level nursing practice. It is designed to test essential nursing knowledge by asking you to apply that knowledge to health care situations demanding nursing intervention.

You are already probably well prepared for such an examination. You have completed a course of instruction in practical nursing. You have learned the basic information necessary to practice safe and effective nursing through various kinds of classroom activities and clinical practice, along with your own study, as determined by each nursing education program's faculty. And you have taken examinations constructed to determine whether or not you have acquired the necessary knowledge and developed an understanding of clinical practice.

That educational process is an excellent preparation for NCLEX-PN. The NCLEX examinations are written by faculty members from nursing education programs around the country, along with clinical practitioners from a wide range of practice areas and settings who supervise recently graduated nurses. Some of your own teachers and clinical supervisors may have been asked, at one time or another, to serve as an item writer for NCLEX-PN.

As to the most basic information about NCLEX-PN, it is a one-day examination given in two time periods of 2½ hours each, one period in the morning and one in the afternoon of each day. During each time period, you are provided one of the two test booklets in which the examination questions are printed and responses are written. There are no separate answer sheets. You are allowed to work only in the booklet provided in each time period. The entire examination consists of about 240 questions.

The examination is given twice a year, in April and October. Scheduled dates through 1999 are provided in the Appendix. All states administer the examination on the same dates but in test sites selected by each state. Many states use more than one test site, with candidates being assigned to regional locations.

Each state board of nursing establishes its own cutoff date for applying for admission to NCLEX and has its own application process with firm deadlines that must be followed by each candidate. You alone are responsible for knowing this information and must request admission to the examination by contacting the board of nursing of the state in which licensure is sought. A list of all the boards of nursing is included in the Appendix.

Following administration of the examination, the test booklets are scored by the National Council's test service. A specific passing point is recommended by the National Council to its Member Boards. However, each state exercises its responsi-

Basic Information

bility to the public by establishing the passing score in its own jurisdiction. Currently, every state has accepted the recommended passing point.

Results are reported to the state board of nursing or other appropriate state agency. It is the state board or agency that will, in turn, notify you of your score.

Preparing for NCLEX-PN

NCLEX-PN is intended to measure the abilities required for practical/vocational nursing practice. What you have learned in nursing school to prepare yourself for practice should provide the necessary preparation for taking NCLEX.

Most candidates will probably want to review in preparation for the examination, and this is appropriate. The best preparation is likely to consist of a review of the textbooks and class notes gathered in nursing school. Later in this introduction, there is an outline of the content covered by NCLEX-PN, which should prove useful in structuring a review of these materials.

What To Study?

In general, it will probably be most helpful for you to study those areas in which you feel least confident, perhaps those areas that caused the most difficulty in nursing school. The questions on NCLEX-PN are designed to test your ability to apply the basic principles of nursing to a wide variety of clinical situations. Therefore, a review of the basic principles of nursing care and their application is suggested.

How To Review?

How you review is, to a large extent, a personal matter, and approaches that have proven successful for you in the past should be relied on again. Along with the nursing knowledge you have gained in your education, you have also learned how to learn and should not underestimate the value of that unique skill.

Reading textbooks and notes is one obvious approach. Another possibility that you may find useful is to study with others preparing to take the examination. Some companionship may be helpful, especially if everyone involved is serious about the work at hand. You can take turns formulating and asking each other questions that serve as a basis for the review.

And, of course, the practice examination presented in this book can be an extremely valuable study tool. The first time you go over these questions, you should answer them as if you were taking the real examination, under quiet conditions and in the same amount of time you will be given. This is an excellent opportunity to get the feel of what it is really like to take NCLEX-PN and to learn the appropriate pace at which you should answer questions. Be sure to time yourself. Check your answers with the answers at the end of the book after you complete the questions.

After the initial use of the questions as a practice examination, the same questions can serve as the basis for a thorough review. Consider each question carefully, especially those you missed. Decide what the question is asking. If you did not answer the question correctly, try to see on your own why the option you chose was not the right one.

In the section where answers are given, there is a brief "rationale" (as it is often called) for the right answer. These brief explanations have been written by clinical practitioners like those who write the questions for NCLEX-PN. Compare your own rationale with those written by these experts. You may be surprised at how much you know. If you know why an answer is correct, consider what other questions could be asked about the nursing situation and how you would answer these further questions. If you do not understand a question, that may indicate a gap in your nursing knowledge, and you will want to go back to your textbooks or study group for review of that topic.

These suggestions are intended as supplements to your study habits, not replacements for them. The fact that you have graduated from an approved school of nursing indicates that you have already developed an extensive set of study skills, and these should serve as the basis for your review for NCLEX-PN.

The amount of time needed for review varies. If you have achieved solid grades in academic and clinical work, then little or no review may be necessary. If you feel you have serious weaknesses in your nursing knowledge, then you may wish to devote several weeks or months to review.

However, regardless of how long your review is, you should schedule it to end a few days before the test date to avoid increasing the anxiety that often accompanies important examinations. It probably is a good idea to watch a movie or engage in some other recreational diversion the night before the test.

The questions on NCLEX-PN emphasize the application of the principles of nursing rather than the recall of facts. By cramming the night before, you may learn a few more facts, but you are unlikely to improve your mastery of the basic principles of nursing. The few facts you acquire probably will not be helpful, and the tension generated by cramming may interfere with your ability to apply what you know to the cases in the examination.

Some students find review courses helpful. If you have developed the basic study skills required in nursing school and have acquired essential nursing knowledge, you should be able to do your review without taking any courses. By working on your own, or with a small group, you can concentrate on those areas of nursing where you feel weakest. But if you feel the need to have your review scheduled and structured for you, a review

How Long To Review?

Are Review Courses Helpful?

4

course may be helpful. In selecting a review course, you should seek one that will provide you with a systematic review of basic nursing.

Many companies have developed diagnostic tools to help candidates for nursing licensure determine their strengths and weaknesses. You may find this type of analysis beneficial for you. Current nursing journals contain advertisements listing these. The nursing school may also give you direction about these diagnostic tools.

Instructions

The first step in taking any examination is to read the instructions very carefully. The instructions for taking the NCLEX-PN are printed in the test booklet and will be read by the proctor at the beginning of the examination period. Pay careful attention to these instructions, and make sure you understand them.

A copy of the instructions that has been used with past examinations is provided with the practice test in this book. A review of these will give you some familiarity with the NCLEX-PN instructions. But be careful—since instructions for NCLEX-PN are revised periodically, instructions in your test booklet could be slightly different from those here. You need to read the instructions in your actual test booklet carefully.

Pace

An important concern in any examination is the pace at which you must work. You are awarded credit for each question that you answer correctly, but you cannot get credit for questions that you have not answered. Some of the questions at the end of the examination may be easier for you than questions that appear earlier. Therefore, you should make sure that you get to the end of the test, and this requires that you pay attention to the time limits.

The schedule for NCLEX-PN has been designed to allow you enough time to answer all the questions. But these time limits assume that you work at a steady pace, about one question per minute, and that you don't spend too much time on any one question or case.

Go through the whole test first, answering those questions for which you can decide on the correct answer in a short time. This will ensure that you get credit for all questions that you can answer easily. On this first run through the test, you should also answer those questions about which you are not sure but think you know the answer. You can return to these doubtful questions later if you have time. Be careful, though. Do not make extra marks in your booklet. With NCLEX-PN, the entire test booklet is scored, and stray marks anywhere in the test booklet could affect your score.

Clinical Situations

NCLEX-PN may be a different kind of examination than you are generally familiar with only because most of the questions on the examination are presented as part of what are called clinical situations. At various points in the examination, a specific clinical situation will be presented. For example:

Sara Anton, 2½ years old, is admitted to the hospital with acute otitis media of the right ear. Her body temperature is elevated.

The information provided in the clinical situation is intended to apply to all questions that appear after the description, so they need to be read as carefully as the questions. It would be helpful to try to visualize the patient as you go through the questions.

Further, more information about the clinical situation may be provided as you make your way through the questions. For example:

Sara's condition improves.

The purpose of this extra information is to make the situation as realistic as possible and to aid you in answering the questions. Don't skip over anything on the examination.

All of the questions on NCLEX-PN are multiple-choice with four answers to choose from. The initial part of a multiple-choice question is called the *stem*, and it is the stem that states the question being asked. The stem is followed by four answers. Only one of these four choices provides the correct answer to the question posed in the stem. The other three choices, which are not correct, are called *distractors*. For example, read the simple question at the right.

In this question, the stem is "A four-month-old is to be weighed daily. At which of the following times would it be best for the nurse to weigh her?" And the correct answer is "Prior to her first morning feeding." The other answers are distractors.

The questions should be read carefully and should be interpreted in a straightforward manner. Do not make assumptions about facts that are not included in the questions or the clinical situations that precede the questions. None of the questions is intended to trick you, and you should try not to "read into" the questions issues that are not there.

The Questions

A four-month-old is to be weighed daily. At which of the following times would it be best for the nurse to weigh her?

○ Prior to her first morning feeding.

○ After she has been bathed.

○ After her first bowel movement of the day.

○ Whenever her mother is available to assist with the procedure.

Strategy

Some nursing educators have expressed a general feeling that candidates who may have difficulty with NCLEX-PN are those who have striven for years to challenge themselves with complex, often tricky intellectual endeavors. Remember, the purpose of NCLEX-PN is not to find the best nurse but to find out who is competent to practice nursing.

In some cases on the examination, the choices for a question may not include the action that you would take in the situation described. In many clinical situations, there are several courses of nursing action that might be appropriate. However, only one of the four choices for each question on NCLEX-PN is correct. If you encounter a question that does not include what you would do in the situation as one of its options, you should imagine yourself doing each of the choices that is listed and decide which is the correct action to take.

It is very important that you try to answer every question. Do not be discouraged if the answer to a question does not come immediately to mind. Most of the questions on the NCLEX-PN require that you apply what you know to the situation described rather than just recognize a fact—and some of the questions are fairly difficult. Therefore, answering the questions requires some thought.

If, after some effort, you still don't know the answer, try to make use of whatever understanding of the problem you do have. For example, even though you might not be sure about what to do in a particular situation, you might know some things not to do. This is valuable information, and you should try to make use of it by eliminating some of the choices from consideration. By limiting your decision to fewer choices, you have improved your chances of picking the correct answer.

There is a practical difference between clinical nursing and test taking. In nursing practice, you shouldn't act on the basis of partial information, vague similarities, and guesses. However, on a test you should indicate what you know, and the fact that your knowledge is incomplete should not stop you from analyzing the question and applying your best judgment. In some cases, your knowledge and judgment may be more complete than you suspect.

This is the question all standardized test-takers ask, and the answer depends on whether or not the examination you are taking is set up with what is called a *correction for guessing*. NCLEX-PN does *not* have a correction for guessing, which means that no points are subtracted for wrong answers. The examination is scored by counting correct answers. Even if you answer with a pure guess, you will have a chance of getting the correct answer.

Should I Guess on NCLEX-PN?

While guessing will not hurt your score, the psychological aspects of guessing remain the same. You will always increase your chances of getting a right answer if you can eliminate one or two choices as being wrong. Guess, but make it educated.

Finally, as you plan for NCLEX-PN, you need to consider what is involved in recording your answers. There is no separate answer sheet for NCLEX-PN. Answers are recorded directly in the test booklet. While this does away with a big danger to any standardized test, losing your place, it does make it necessary to require that no stray marks be written in the test booklet. Do not use the booklet for scratch paper or notes to yourself.

The example at the right shows how questions appear in the test booklet.

Use only a number 2 pencil and fill in completely the circle next to the answer you choose, being careful to erase completely any stray marks or responses you wish to change.

Foreign-educated nurses have much to contribute to health care in this country. After all, the United States has always embraced a diversity of nationalities. Your special outlook and experiences as a foreign-educated nurse can be an advantage as long as your education has provided you with skills equivalent to those of nursing candidates from U.S. programs.

The main purpose of the licensure examination is to protect the public. Passing the licensing examination in effect states that you are capable of delivering safe and effective nursing care to the public in the United States regardless of where you were educated. The diversity and welcome variation that you, as a foreign-educated nurse, bring to the public must be considered *after* you have given evidence of your ability to deliver effective health care. For you, the licensure examination is particularly important.

You may have several major questions about qualifying to practice nursing in the United States. This book focuses upon the licensure examination you must take and pass. Other questions about licensure or qualifications to take the licensure examination, such as passing an English test or the Commission on Graduates of Foreign Nursing Schools examination can be sent to the state board of nursing in the state in which you wish to practice. A list of boards of nursing and their addresses is provided in the Appendix.

This book describes the type of examination you will take and gives you a sample test. The questions are all multiple-choice. The chapters of this book on how to review for the test should also be studied.

Steve Holmes, 8 years old, has sickle cell anemia. He is admitted to the hospital in sickle cell crisis.

---

1. Steve complains of pain in his legs and abdomen. The nurse should understand that such pain is probably the result of
   ○ bleeding into the cellular spaces.
   ○ clumping of erythrocytes.
   ○ a generalized infectious process.
   ○ a shift of intestinal fluid.

Foreign-Educated Nurses

Review courses may also give some assistance. If, after reviewing the sample test in this book, you find you are unfamiliar with this type of testing and wish additional assistance, you can select a review course offered by a local college near you or by an independent organization. Courses on how to take a multiple-choice test may be particularly helpful if you have not taken this kind of test before.

Diagnostic tools to help you define areas of strengths and weaknesses may also help. The state board of nursing and nursing journals will give you information about specific diagnostic tests that you might use.

Role of Cultural Differences

You may also wonder if nursing is somewhat different in the United States. According to studies on this subject, you may find a somewhat different emphasis here than in the country where you were educated. Cultural differences may have some impact on your perception of patient needs. The section of this introduction describing the content of the examination and what sample questions are testing should help you determine if this will be a problem for you. In addition, after trying the sample examination in this book, review each question and correct answer to determine if cultural differences may have had an impact on your choice of answers.

If you find this is a problem, review with United States-educated nurses or faculty to try to understand the attitudes of people here in the United States to whom you will be expected to give care. Being able to give safe and effective care to people from a cultural background different from yours may be a problem for you; it should not be made the problem of the person seeking help—the client. Again, courses in local colleges may be of some assistance.

Reading Level of NCLEX-PN

Besides the possibility of cultural differences, if you do not know English well, you may be worried about the reading difficulty of the licensure examination. Those who participate in developing the examination are aware of the need to keep the reading difficulty as low as possible. There are terms used in health care fields that nurses are supposed to know and these are used. Nontechnical words are reviewed with the understanding that the test is not a test of reading ability. Vocabulary is made as easy as possible. The estimated reading level of the examination is the 8th grade. To understand what this means, compare this practice examination to nursing textbooks in English. Most of the current nursing textbooks are at the 12th grade reading level. If you find that you can understand the language used in the textbooks without difficulty, probably you will not find the level of reading in the examination difficult.

Of course, the best check on the reading level of the examination is to look at the test questions contained in this book. If the wording of many questions is difficult for you, your proficiency in English may be a problem in taking the licensure examination.

The other suggestions contained in this book for preparing for the examination can be used by you, as well as by candidates who have completed a nursing program in the United States. The suggestions for study are valuable for all candidates. Generally, additional information on extra assistance by tutors, classes, etc., can be obtained through the state board of nursing located in the state in which you plan to practice nursing.

The Process of Developing NCLEX-PN

Examination Committee

The National Council has placed responsibility for the development of the licensure examinations in its Examination Committee, which is composed of individuals who are either board members or staff members selected from Member Boards of Nursing. There are representatives of the four regions of the country—West, South, Midwest, and Northeast—on the committee at all times.

A flow chart depicting the process of developing an NCLEX examination is given in the Appendix. As you can see, the members of the Examination Committee prepare what is called a test plan for the examination—one for NCLEX-PN and one for NCLEX-RN.

Test Plan

The test plan is an outline of the nursing content to be covered on NCLEX, based on studies of current nursing practice. As a professional licensure examination, NCLEX must test a candidate's professional capabilities for a first-time, or entry-level, position. It is not intended to test achievement in nursing school, or to require the professional experience of nurses who have worked for several years. The entry level of nursing capability is determined through periodic studies of the jobs that entry-level nurses are actually performing throughout the United States.

From the information collected in these studies, the Examination Committee constructs a test plan. The test plan is then submitted to the National Council's Delegate Assembly, comprised of representatives from each of its Member Boards, for its approval.

Item Writers

Following approval of the test plan, the Member Boards on a rotating basis are invited to submit names of persons to write test questions. These people are referred to as item writers and may be faculty members from associate degree, diploma, and baccalaureate programs, or clinical nurse specialists who have contact with students or beginning practitioners. The National Council's Examination Committee selects groups of item writers

10

yearly on the basis of their credentials, the region of the country they represent, the type of nursing program they represent, and their expertise in nursing.

The selected item writers work for a week with the staff of the test service to develop new questions. Common clinical situations are chosen, each of which may yield a series of questions. The questions are checked by the test service following each item-writing session to make certain that questions meet examination specifications, are not ethnically or sexually biased, and are grammatically correct. Both the clinically expert item writers on hand at the session, and current nursing textbooks and journals, must support the intended correct answer.

Review of New Questions

After the items are written, a Panel of Content Experts will review the new questions to determine that each is accurate, current, related to the job of the entry-level nurse, and that the answer chosen is in fact correct. Members of the panel are chosen in much the same way as item writers, by the National Council's Examination Committee from nominations submitted annually by Member Boards on a rotating basis. These nurses are not faculty members. They are clinical practitioners who work directly with entry-level nurses.

Member Boards may also request to review the proposed items. Boards focus their determinations on how consistent the questions are with nursing practice in their state as defined by their laws and regulations, and if it reflects entry-level practice.

Testing New Questions

These newly developed questions are then placed in actual NCLEX examinations and answered by actual candidates. These do not count toward passing or failing the examination. Your natural reaction might be to worry about having to answer trial questions, but don't be concerned that the time you spend on a try-out question might be taking away from time you need to spend on a real question. The examination has been planned to allow you ample time to answer both real questions and trial questions.

Answer every question carefully because there is a need for practical information from you about the newly developed test questions to make sure they are written clearly and are relevant to practical/vocational nursing practice. Obtaining responses on trial questions in this way ensures that the nursing content being tested is current in all states and not confined to selected regions. If there is a trend toward a different emphasis in practical/vocational nurse practice in one region of the country, it will be reflected in responses to the try-out questions.

Data from the trial questions can also identify sources of ambiguity by indicating questions for which a large number of candidates pick the same wrong answer. Even though questions are thoroughly reviewed before they are included as trial questions, occasionally you may interpret a question in a way that was not intended when it was written.

Statistical analyses of the trial questions are reviewed by the test service staff. Questions that do not meet the statistical guideline set by the Examination Committee are not used in future examinations.

This system of checks and balances is used to ensure that only questions testing essential knowledge are used. Every effort is made to ensure that the questions are clear and relevant, and test important content. There are no trick questions; there are no questions with double meanings; there are no unanswerable questions.

You may wonder about the currency of the licensure examination. Many times people assume that a period of several years occurs between the selection of test content and the administration of the examinations. The Panel of Content Experts has currency as the major focus for its review of questions. Also, the Examination Committee members, with the assistance of the test service staff, select the questions to be used in each of the examinations only a short time before the examinations are given. Currency of content is a continuing concern. The short time between selection and administration assures that the NCLEX examinations are kept current.

Currency of Licensure Examinations

Now that you are familiar with the way in which individual questions are written, you may be curious about the test plan itself and how it came to be.

The NCLEX-PN Test Plan

Until 1982, the nursing licensure examinations used by boards of nursing throughout the United States were called the State Board Test Pool Examinations for Registered Nurses and Practical Nurses (SBTPE-RN and SBTPE-PN). The test plan upon which the SBTPE-PN was based, in use since 1952, was devised as a result of a survey in which experts responded to questions concerning what practical/vocational nursing was or ought to be. Although the test plan underwent some editing and modification to reflect changes in nursing, the basic form remained unchanged until implementation of a new test plan in 1985.

The 1985 test plan was based on a study that updated nursing's knowledge of the current role of entry-level practical/vocational nurses by identifying the actual job activities performed by the entry-level practical/vocational nurses. The study also compared those activities to the activities tested by the NCLEX-PN test plan. The study entitled *Practical Nurse Role Delineation and Validation Study for the National Council Licensure Examination for Practical Nurses,* was performed by the National Council's test service, CTB/McGraw-Hill, under leadership of Helen M. Ference, Ph.D., R.N.

The current test plan is based on information gathered from newly licensed practical/vocational nurses in 1986 and 1987. The results of this job analysis study is entitled *Job Analysis of Newly Licensed Practical/Vocational Nurses (1986-87)*.

The test plan for the NCLEX-PN is divided into four client need categories based on the steps of the nursing process. A copy of the test plan is given in the Appendix. Referring to it will help you understand the following examples of questions:

How Questions Fit the Test Plan

Category I—Collecting Data: contributes to the development of a client's data base.

A client is scheduled for an intravenous pyelogram. Which of the following information is important for the nurse to obtain from the client before this procedure is done?
① 24-hour urine output.
② Thyroid functioning.
③ History of allergies.
④ Adequacy of bowel evacuation.

In order to respond correctly to the situation described above, you need to know that the assessment of allergies to iodine-based compounds is essential before a client has an IVP. The correct answer is #3.

Category II—Planning: contributes to the development of the client's nursing care plan.

A client is admitted with gangrene of the left foot. In order to prevent further tissue breakdown, the nurse should plan to use which of the following?
① Sheepskin pad.
② Heat lamp.
③ Bed board.
④ Bed cradle.

In this second example, to arrive at the correct answer, #4, you must be able to recognize symptoms and plan the appropriate nursing care.

13

Category III—Implementing: performing and recording nursing care given by following a prescribed plan of care.

A client has organic brain syndrome. The nurse finds the client standing near the bathroom door. The client has wet herself, as she does occasionally, because she does not allow herself sufficient time to reach the bathroom. The client looks ashamed and turns away from the nurse. Which of the following responses by the nurse would be **best**?

① "Can you tell me why you waited so long to go to the bathroom?"
② "I know that this is upsetting to you. Come with me and I'll get a change of clothes for you."
③ "Can you think of any way in which we can help you to manage your bathroom trips?"
④ "Go to your room and change your dirty clothes."

The correct response to the third example is #2. This requires knowledge of communication skills in order to intervene with the appropriate response.

Category IV—Evaluating: assists in evaluating the effectiveness of the client's nursing care and making appropriate alterations to that care.

The nurse asks a client to select foods that best meet her low-fat, low-sodium diet prescription. In evaluating the client's knowledge of her diet, the nurse would expect the client to choose which of the following menus?

① Tossed salad with blue cheese dressing, cold cuts, and vanilla cookies.
② Split pea soup, cheese sandwich, and a banana.
③ Cold baked chicken, lettuce with salad tomatoes, and applesauce.
④ Beans and frankfurters, carrot and celery sticks, and a plain cupcake.

The final example tests your ability to evaluate the client's knowledge of her diet. The correct answer is #3.

If you refer to the test plan in the Appendix, you can see that there are four categories of client needs which require actions by nurses. These categories are:

1. *Safe, effective care environment.* This broad category considers clients' needs for environmental safety, care

that is goal-oriented and coordinated, and measures that assure quality and safety.

2. *Physiological integrity.* The nurse's consideration of needs of the clients contained under this category include physiological adaptation, reduction of risk, mobility, comfort, and basic care.

3. *Psychosocial integrity.* Psychosocial integrity in stress and crisis-related situations necessitates actions by the nurse that emphasize client adaptation.

4. *Health promotion/maintenance.* Self-care and growth and development are major client needs considered in this category. Also, client needs related to the prevention of diseases and assurance of integrity of support systems require nursing actions that are classified here.

The question under Category I of the nursing process is an example of client safety which is part of safe, effective care environment. Obtaining general client information about allergies is also addressed in this situation.

An example of physiological integrity is seen in the question under Category II. The nurse is involved in risk reduction and comfort behavior.

Psychosocial integrity is demonstrated by the question under Category III. The nurse, using communication skills, is helping the client cope and adapt to her situation.

The question under Category IV is an example of the nurse assisting the client with self-care behaviors.

Background and Technical Information for the Licensure Examination

Nursing licensure examinations were initiated in 1944. At that time they were called the State Board Test Pool Examinations (SBTPE). The title was changed to National Council Licensure Examination in 1981. The examinations evolved during the years between 1933 and 1950 when cooperative agreements between two major organizations—the American Nurses' Association and the National League of Nursing Education (later the National League for Nursing)—were made to assist the state boards of nurse examiners.

The state boards were responsible for developing and administering a licensing examination for nursing, and they were under pressure to increase the validity and reliability of examinations, as well as to hasten the scoring time. Because of World War II and the resulting need for nurses, it was necessary to streamline the licensing process and yet maintain a valid examination to protect the public from unsafe health care practitioners.

However, even prior to World War II, the need to produce examinations that accurately tested nursing competence had united the state boards of nurse examiners in their efforts to develop a uniform national examination.

Four states participated in the first administration of the State Board Test Pool Examination for Registered Nurses in January 1944. By the middle of 1944, 15 states were using the newly developed tests. By 1950, all 48 states and the District of Columbia were participating in the SBTPE-RN. Since that time, Alaska, Hawaii, Guam, the Virgin Islands, American Samoa, and the Commonwealth of Northern Mariana Islands have initiated use of the examination.

The SBTPE-PN was first used in 1948, however not all states adopted its use until 1962. Texas used the examination in the early 1950s, but it was not used on a continuous basis until 1968. California used SBTPE-PN through 1974, but discontinued its use until 1986 when that state began using NCLEX-PN.

Currently, the National Council of State Boards of Nursing, who develop NCLEX, maintains a liaison with the organizations that represent practical/vocational nursing: the National Association for Practical Nurse Education and Service and the National Federation of Licensed Practical Nurses. In addition, many licensed practical nurses have been appointed to state boards of nurse examiners and provide input to the licensure examination.

How NCLEX-PN Is Administered and Scored

NCLEX-PN contains about 240 questions and is given in two parts, called Books I and II for ease in administering the examination and to provide a break during the one day of testing. These parts do not differ from each other in subject area covered. You will be given a pass/fail result for the entire examination, not a separate result for each book.

The basic purpose of a licensure examination is to determine if a person is competent to practice. All effort is expended to do this. Therefore, it is consistent to report that you have the knowledge, skills, and abilities to provide safe care (pass) or that you do not demonstrate the knowledge, skills, and abilities to practice nursing (fail).

Formerly, the licensure examinations were scored on what is called a norm-referenced system. A norm-referenced system calculates each score in comparison to a norming population; that is, each score is interpreted in comparison to the group of scores of all the candidates taking an examination at the same time. An example of norm-referenced testing is: if the questions in a test are difficult for the group, a score of 30 could represent a high level of achievement; if the questions are easy for the group, a score of 30 could represent a low level of achievement.

The National Council decided to go to a criterion-referenced scoring system in 1982. With a criterion referenced scoring system, a "criterion" or standard judged to represent an acceptable level of competence is set. That is, a minimum score is set to guarantee that a candidate who demonstrates a certain level of nursing knowledge passes the test. In the remote possibility that an entire group of candidates did very well on the examination, they could all be given passing scores. In practice, however, it should be quickly added that the current pass/fail rate has not changed appreciably with the change to a criterion-referenced system. In essence, the criterion-referenced system simply provides a safeguard against admitting incompetent candidates to the nursing profession because the test is scored against a standard that represents minimum competence requirements.

You may be worried, as you read this, about how this minimum level of competence is determined, and how the National Council assures that the lowest passing score is arrived at fairly. This is a complicated issue, involving a combination of the judgment of nursing experts together with statistical techniques.

The National Council uses a standard-setting process known as the Angoff method, a commonly used criterion-referenced, standard-setting technique. This method depends on a panel of expert judges who review the test questions on the examination. The National Council uses this method because it is a relatively straightforward procedure that tends to yield a reasonable standard. The procedure involves four steps:

1. The selection and convening of a panel of at least nine judges who are current nursing practitioners who work directly with or supervise entry-level nurses.

2. Definition of lowest acceptable level of performance is determined. This is done through training of the judges by the test service staff. The judges, working together, agree on the characteristics of a minimally competent beginning nurse.

3. Independent judgment of the performance of a minimally competent candidate on all questions in the examination. This step involves each judge taking a copy of the examination and reviewing it question by

question, rating each question on the probability that a minimally competent candidate can answer it correctly.

4. Aggregation of the judgments to produce a passing score for the examination. In this step, all judges' estimates for each question will be averaged. The judges may discuss significant discrepancies among themselves. The averages for all questions are then added together to yield the criterion-referenced standard for the examination.

To illustrate this procedure, you can compare the panel of judges to a group of faculty responsible for a course in nursing. First, they define course objectives. Then, they determine the essential knowledge, skills, and abilities that the students must demonstrate to pass the course. Because of the variability in student performance on paper and pencil tests, faculty average the results of all tests. The faculty also discuss among themselves and reconcile any issues on which they are divided.

Candidate Diagnostic Profile

You are right if you feel that this process depends heavily on individual subjective judgments and not simply on ''impartial'' statistical techniques. It does depend on the personal judgments of the panel of experts, as does an examination given by an individual instructor in a nursing course. However, this standard-setting process also involves statistical techniques that help to individualize decisions. Also the results of the panel, along with other relevant data, is reviewed by the National Council's Board of Directors in setting a passing score. The National Council believes this method is the most appropriate to make sure that nurses about to enter practice are competent and safe in the delivery of care to patients.

Candidate Diagnostic Profile

For those candidates who fail NCLEX-PN, the results can be painful enough without the added frustration that comes with not knowing as much as possible about why the failure occurred.

To provide information that can help a licensure candidate focus review efforts in preparation for retaking the examination, the National Council's Examination Committee developed the NCLEX Candidate Diagnostic Profile to accompany each failing candidate's score report.

As the reproduction of the Diagnostic Profile, both front and back, indicates, it is an outline based on the NCLEX-PN test plan. Each question on an examination is coded according to the test plan classifications.

The NCLEX Diagnostic Profile diagrams failing candidates' performance on a scale that extends from low to high. You will note that a legend in the bottom right-hand corner tells you about how many questions you missed passing by. The profile also tells you how well you performed in each test plan category. This will aid you in determining which areas of the test plan you need to study the most.

Statistical Background

Although this explanation of passing and failing NCLEX-PN seems straightforward enough, you should be aware that sophisticated statistical methods are required to be sure that your results are calculated fairly and that the test accurately measures what it is intended to measure.

Here again, the National Council depends on its test service. The test service is responsible for considering two important statistical factors that determine whether a test is a good one: its validity and its reliability.

The validity of the results has to do with the test's accuracy— in the case of NCLEX, does it really measure whether you can be a safe, effective, entry-level nurse? The reliability of results has to do with its consistency—in the case of NCLEX, if you took the examination again would you get the same results? Or, to put it another way, if the practical nursing examination is valid and reliable, adequately prepared practical/vocational nurses will pass it, and, if they take it over and over, they will get the same result each time.

Conclusion

The purpose of this book is to explain the background and development of the licensure examination for practical/ vocational nursing. It gives questions so that you may have first-hand knowledge of the type of questions you will see on the examination. The information throughout is given to help you understand what knowledge, skills, and ability you will need to demonstrate in order to be successful in the examination. Many times approaching something totally unknown makes it an object of fear. The intent here is to reduce the unknown so that you may demonstrate that you are competent to give safe, effective, entry-level nursing care.

NCLEX CANDIDATE DIAGNOSTIC PROFILE
National Council Licensure Examination for Practical Nurses

Candidate Number:
Date of Birth:
Social Security Number:

The location of the "**X**" on the first diagram below is based upon your overall performance on the NCLEX examination. Directly below the "**X**" is a symbol. Check the legend in the lower right-hand corner to see by how many items you missed the passing point. The "**X**"s on the subsequent diagrams, which relate to the categories in the NCLEX-PN Test Plan, represent your level of performance on the items testing the knowledge, skills, and abilities essential for performing each job dimension indicated. (Detailed information regarding the percentage of questions on the examination from each of these test plan areas is included on the reverse side of this form.) The gray, shaded bars in the test plan area boxes are given as a reference point only. (Since the test plan areas are not subtests, you do not "pass" or "fail" in these areas. If your performance were to exceed the reference point ( ) in each test plan area, you would be certain to pass the exam.) You are advised not only to review general nursing content, but to concentrate your review on the categories where your "**X**" is farthest from the reference point.

Overall Performance Assessment

| = PASSING POINT

X
low performance   **|**   high performance

#

PHASES OF THE NURSING PROCESS*

Data Collection

X
low performance   high performance

Planning

X
low performance   high performance

Implementation

X
low performance   high performance

Evaluation

X
low performance   high performance

CATEGORIES OF CLIENT NEEDS*

Safe, Effective Care Environment

X
low performance   high performance

Physiological Integrity

X
low performance   high performance

Psychosocial Integrity

X
low performance   high performance

Health Promotion/Maintenance

X
low performance   high performance

LEGEND for Overall Performance Assessment Diagram
Missed passing by:
¢ = 12 or fewer questions
+ = 13-24 questions
@ = 25-36 questions
# = 37 or more questions

*Note: Definitions and information regarding percentages of questions in each test plan category are printed on the reverse side of this report.

NATIONAL COUNCIL

20

Definitions

PHASES OF THE NURSING PROCESS

The phases of the nursing process are described as follows:

I. Collecting Data (30% of an examination)
   A. Contribute to the development of a database.
   B. Participate in the formulation of nursing diagnoses.

II. Planning (20% of an examination)
   A. Contribute to the development of nursing care plans.
   B. Assist in the formulation of goals.
   C. Participate in the identification of clients' needs and nursing measures required to achieve goals.
   D. Communicate needs that may require alteration of the care plan.
   E. Communicate with the client, significant others, and/or health team members in planning nursing care.

III. Implementing (30% of an examination)
   A. Perform basic therapeutic and preventive nursing measures by following a prescribed plan of care to achieve established client goals.
   B. Provide a safe and effective environment.
   C. Assist client, significant others, and health care members to understand the client's plan of care.
   D. Record client information and report it to other health team members.

IV. Evaluating (20% of an examination)
   A. Participate in evaluating the effectiveness of the client's nursing care.
   B. Assist in evaluating the client's response to nursing care and in making appropriate alterations.
   C. Evaluate the extent to which identified outcomes of the care plan are achieved.
   D. Record and describe client's responses to therapy and/or care.

CATEGORIES OF CLIENT NEEDS

The categories of client needs are described as follows:

I. Safe, Effective Care Environment (24% to 30% of an examination)

This category includes the client needs listed below:

   1. Coordinated care
   2. Quality assurance
   3. Goal-oriented care
   4. Environmental safety
   5. Preparation for treatments and procedures
   6. Safe and effective treatments and procedures

The following are examples of areas in which the nurse should possess the knowledge, skills, and abilities necessary to meet these needs:

Data-gathering techniques; interpersonal communication skills; alternative methods of communication for clients with special needs; client preparation for prescribed treatments and procedures; environmental and client safety; infection control; client rights; confidentiality; individualization of care, including religious, cultural, and developmental influences; team participation in care planning; and evaluation and general knowledge of community agencies.

CATEGORIES OF CLIENT NEEDS (continued)

II. Physiological Integrity (42% to 48% of an examination)

This category includes the client needs listed below:
   7. Physiological adaptation
   8. Reduction of risk potential
   9. Mobility
   10. Comfort
   11. Provision of basic care

The following are examples of areas in which the nurse should possess the knowledge, skills, and abilities necessary to meet these needs:

Therapeutic and life-saving procedures, specialized equipment, principles of administering medications, maintenance of optimal body functioning and prevention of complications, principles of body mechanics and assistive devices, comfort measures, routine nursing measures, and reporting changes in a client's condition.

III. Psychosocial Integrity (7% to 13% of an examination)

This category includes the client needs listed below:
   12. Psychosocial adaptation
   13. Coping/Adaptation

The following are examples of areas in which the nurse should possess the knowledge, skills, and abilities necessary to meet these needs:

Obvious signs of emotional and mental health problems, self-concept, life crises, chemical dependency, adaptive and maladaptive behavior, sensory deprivation and overload, abusive and self-destructive behavior, therapeutic communication, common therapies, and general knowledge of community resources.

IV. Health Promotion/Maintenance (15% to 21% of an examination)

This category includes the client needs listed below:
   14. Continued growth and development
   15. Self-care
   16. Integrity of support system
   17. Prevention and early treatment of disease

The following are examples of areas in which the nurse should possess the knowledge, skills, and abilities necessary to meet these needs:

Family interactions; concepts of wellness; adaptation to altered health states; reproduction and human sexuality; birthing and parenting; growth and development, including dying and death; immunization; health teaching that is appropriate to the scope of practice; and general knowledge of community resources.

Specific definitions for the Test Plan Categories are included in the Test Plan for the National Council Licensure Examination for Practical Nurses. To order this Test Plan, send a $3.00 check or money order to the National Council of State Boards of Nursing, Inc., 676 N. St. Clair, Suite 550, Chicago, IL 60611.

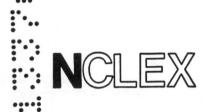

NCLEX

The National Council Licensure Examination
for Practical Nurses

Form 787–A

Part I

Last Name   **First Name**   **Middle Name**

Birth Date

____ / ____ / ____
month   day   year

Signature

_____

Place your admission card here. Align arrows. Copy your candidate number in the boxes below exactly as it appears on your admission card. Carefully fill in the appropriate circle below each digit.

Your Candidate Number

The following information will be used to perform certain statistical analyses of the test questions. Providing this information is voluntary and failure to do so will have no effect on your score. Information obtained concerning individuals will be kept confidential.

Fill in the circle that applies to you.

○ White   ○ Asian Indian
○ Black   ○ Other Asian
○ American Indian ○ Hispanic
○ Pacific Islander ○ Other

Fill in the circle that applies to you.

○ Male
○ Female

Published by CTB/McGraw-Hill

74249

This is Part I of the National Council Licensure Examination, which consists of two parts. Each part is in a separate booklet and consists of approximately 120 questions. Included here are some suggestions to help you do your best on this examination. Each question lists four possible answers. You are to select only one answer for each question. Read each question carefully before you decide which one of the suggested answers is correct. Press firmly on your pencil and darken the circle completely next to your answer choice in the examination booklet. You **MUST** use a No. 2 pencil to mark your answers. Erase any stray marks on the page as the examination will be scored by machine and stray marks may be interpreted as incorrect answers. Do not bend or fold any part of the booklet. Use the page identified as "NOTES" for any calculations or notes you might want to make.

The following is a sample question with the correct answer marked properly.

1   Rose, 2 years old, is to receive an antibiotic orally
in liquid form. Before pouring the medication,
it is essential for the nurse to do which of
the following?

○ wipe the lid with a sterile cotton ball
○ hold the bottle under warm water
○ ask if Rose has ever taken liquid medications
● shake the bottle well

The fourth choice is the correct answer, and the circle next to it has been marked.

When marking your answer, darken only one circle for each question. Darken the circle completely. Do NOT use X's or check marks. If you decide to change your answer, erase your original answer thoroughly. If you do not, your new answer may be scored incorrectly. Also erase all stray marks on the page. You **MUST** use a No. 2 pencil to mark your answers.

Incorrect Marks   **Correct Mark**

○   ○   ○   ○   ○

○   ○   ○   ○   ○

◉   ◑   ⓧ   ☑   ●

○   ○   ○   ○   ○

To do your best on this examination, be sure that you understand the following directions before beginning the examination.

• Read each question carefully.

• Select the correct answer from the four possible choices.

• There is only one correct answer to each question.

• Work in a systematic manner; do not spend too much time on any one question.

• If the answer you might prefer is not included, choose one of those listed. Any question that is not answered will be scored as incorrect.

Follow these directions carefully.

DO NOT TURN THE PAGE UNTIL TOLD TO DO SO

I-3

23

The National Council Licensure Examination for Practical Nurses

PART I

**You will be allowed 2 hours
to complete this part of the examination.**

Please begin.

Mr. Morris Samm, a 48-year-old married man, has been using nitroglycerin tablets for several months for relief of angina pectoris.

1. Which of the following observations made by the nurse would relate to Mr. Samm's diagnosis of angina pectoris?

① He experiences shortness of breath when climbing stairs.

② He is very lethargic after eating an unusually heavy meal.

③ His fingers are numb and tingle when he is relaxed and resting.

④ He complains of sudden pain in the substernal region after a disagreement with his wife.

2. The nurse should understand that the desired effect from Mr. Samm's nitroglycerin is to

① constrict his peripheral blood vessels.

② improve his coronary blood flow.

③ produce slower and stronger heartbeats.

④ increase the rate and depth of respirations.

Mr. Samm has attacks of severe chest pain that are not relieved by the nitroglycerin. He is admitted to the hospital with a myocardial infarction. Complete bed rest, oxygen by nasal cannula, anticoagulant therapy, a low-sodium diet, and morphine sulfate are prescribed for him.

3. Mr. Samm had morphine one hour before morning care is given. When the nurse attempts to turn Mr. Samm, he lies absolutely still, refuses to move, and holds his left shoulder with his hand. The nurse interprets this behavior to mean that Mr. Samm

① finds this the most comfortable position.

② is protecting himself from his surroundings.

③ fears that the pain will recur.

④ is indicating that he is chilly.

4. To promote safety while Mr. Samm is receiving oxygen, which of the following precautions should the nurse take?

① Be sure the room is well ventilated.

② Keep electrical equipment to a minimum.

③ Increase the humidity level of the room.

④ Post no smoking signs around the room.

5. While Mr. Samm is receiving the oral anticoagulant, the nurse should observe him for evidence of

① hives.

② difficulty in breathing.

③ restlessness.

④ hematuria.

6. While Mr. Samm is on a low-sodium diet, the nurse should encourage him to select which of the following foods?

① Cereals and dairy products.

② Bakery products and processed meats.

③ Fresh vegetables and fruits.

④ Canned soups and grains.

7. Which of these questions should the nurse give greatest consideration to in selecting a diversion for Mr. Samm?

① Will it be new to him?

② Will it amuse him?

③ Does it promote relaxation?

④ Does it require mental concentration?

8. Mr. Samm is a Roman Catholic. His wife says to the nurse, "I want my husband to be anointed, but I don't want to frighten him." Which of these responses by the nurse would be most appropriate?

① "Would you like to talk with a priest about this?"

② "This is a decision you must make yourself."

③ "Perhaps your husband isn't nearly as frightened as you are about death."

④ "If I were you, I wouldn't bring the matter up at this time unless your husband mentions it himself."

9. If Mr. Samm's pulse is described as being thready, which characteristics would the nurse observe?

① Slow and irregular.

② Slow and forceful.

③ Rapid and weak.

④ Rapid and bounding.

10. Which signs would the nurse observe if Mr. Samm developed Cheyne-Stokes respirations?

① Stertorous, deep, labored breathing.

② Shallow respirations, gradually increasing in rate.

③ Gradually increasing dyspnea and rapid, deep respirations.

④ Alternating periods of irregular breathing and apnea.

11. Mr. Samm dies. Which of the following nursing actions are necessary in caring for the body after death?

① Padding body prominences.

② Keeping the body in a side-lying position.

③ Positioning the body to prevent drainage from the orifices.

④ Handling the body to protect it from disfigurement.

12. Which of the following would be **most** important to include in Ms. Miller's nursing care plan?

① Restriction of food and fluids.

② Observation of amount and type of vaginal drainage.

③ Instructions on birth control measures.

④ Limitation of activity until pain and bleeding cease.

Ms. Miller is scheduled to have a dilatation and curettage (D and C) the next day. Her preoperative prescriptions include secobarbital (Seconal) at bedtime.

---

13. In addition to promoting sleep, the nurse should understand that Seconal is given to Ms. Miller for which of these purposes?

① To reduce the level of anxiety.

② To lessen bronchial secretions.

③ To decrease the muscle tone of the uterus.

④ To minimize the need for postoperative analgesia.

14. When checking Ms. Miller's chart on the morning of surgery, the nurse finds that there is no operative consent. Which of these actions should the nurse take **first**?

① Obtain an operative consent form and have Ms. Miller sign it.

② Report the absence of an operative consent to the registered nurse in charge.

③ Notify the operating room staff that the operative consent has not been obtained.

④ Ask Ms. Miller whether she signed an operative consent form on admission to the hospital.

GO ON TO THE NEXT PAGE.

15. Ms. Miller receives meperidine hydrochloride (Demerol) and atropine sulfate preoperatively. Which of the following should the nurse recognize as the expected outcome of these medications?

① The effectiveness of the anesthesia was increased.

② There was no postoperative dehydration.

③ The tone of smooth muscle was improved, thus preventing hemorrhage.

④ The respiratory secretions were reduced during surgery.

Ms. Miller has a D and C under general anesthesia. She is conscious when she is brought back to her unit.

---

16. Blood work drawn during surgery is reported to the unit. Ms. Miller's red blood count is 2,500,000 per cu. mm. of blood. Which of the following actions should the nurse take?

① Notify the registered nurse in charge of the results.

② Force fluids to 3,000 cc per 24 hours.

③ Encourage Ms. Miller to rest as much as possible.

④ Continue with Ms. Miller's established plan of care.

17. An iron preparation is prescribed for Ms. Miller. The nurse should administer the iron preparation at which of these times?

① Immediately before breakfast.

② Between meals.

③ Immediately after meals.

④ At bedtime.

Mr. Samuel Gayle, 42 years old, has chronic lymphocytic leukemia. Mr. Gayle has been told that his condition is terminal. He takes an antiemetic prn at home. Mr. Gayle has come to the clinic to receive a blood transfusion for anemia.

18. The nurse should understand that Mr. Gayle may display which of the following symptoms typical of a patient with chronic lymphocytic leukemia?

① Weakness and fatigue.

② Pain in the joints and dizziness.

③ Confusion and tachycardia.

④ Dyspnea and headache.

19. Prior to the blood transfusion, Mr. Gayle is given diphenhydramine hydrochloride (Benadryl). The nurse recognizes that the purpose of this measure is to

① sedate him for the transfusion.

② prevent hemolysis of the blood.

③ permit a more rapid infusion of the blood.

④ minimize a possible transfusion reaction.

20. Mr. Gayle complains of a bad taste in his mouth from bleeding gums. Which of the following measures would be **most** important for the nurse to include in Mr. Gayle's care plan?

① Suck on hard candy or chew gum to relieve the bad taste.

② Use a soft bristle toothbrush and rinse his mouth frequently with normal saline.

③ Floss teeth and rinse his mouth frequently with mouthwash.

④ Drink cold beverages and use lemon-glycerin swabs.

21. Mr. Gayle complains of nausea and anorexia. Which of these suggestions by the nurse would **best** promote Mr. Gayle's food intake?

① Mr. Gayle should eat at regular mealtimes and save uneaten food for between-meal feedings.

② Mr. Gayle should eat foods high in protein and drink high nitrogen liquid supplements.

③ Mr. Gayle should take his antiemetic a half hour before meals and eat a diet of small, bland feedings.

④ Mr. Gayle should eat what he can during meals and not worry about the rest.

GO ON TO THE NEXT PAGE.

22. Mr. Gayle has been depressed since the physician told him that his condition is terminal. Which of the following approaches should the nurse include in the care plan?

① Ignore Mr. Gayle's depression.

② Accept Mr. Gayle's depression.

③ Counterbalance Mr. Gayle's depression.

④ Challenge Mr. Gayle's depression.

23. Mr. Gayle says to the nurse, "The doctor told me that my blood condition is too severe to be treated successfully. This probably means that I don't have long to live." Which of the following responses would be **most** appropriate for the nurse to make?

① "Your condition is serious, Mr. Gayle."

② "You should be thinking about making out a will, Mr. Gayle."

③ "It would be better for you to think of something else, Mr. Gayle."

④ "There is always hope, Mr. Gayle."

24. The physician tells Mr. Gayle to use acetaminophen (Tylenol) rather than aspirin for any pain. In preparing Mr. Gayle for discharge, the nurse should explain

① Tylenol is more effective than aspirin in controlling the pain caused by his disease.

② Tylenol is absorbed in the stomach more rapidly than aspirin, thus relieving pain more quickly.

③ aspirin interferes with prothrombin formation causing more potential for bleeding.

④ aspirin requires more frequent dosages, thus increasing the danger of toxicity.

25. While the nurse is preparing June's leg for the biopsy, June says, "If this lump turns out to be cancer, what happens next?" Which of the following responses would be **most** appropriate for the nurse to make?

① "I can't say. It's really hard to know exactly what will happen."

② "I know you're worried. Have you spoken with your doctor about it?"

③ "What makes you think that you might have cancer?"

④ "It's best to wait until after the biopsy to find out if it's cancer."

The biopsy is performed and the results indicate that a malignancy is present. The physician informs June and her parents of the results of the biopsy. June is hospitalized and scheduled for a below-the-knee amputation of her right leg.

26. At 2 a.m. on the morning of surgery, the nurse finds June awake and crying. In addition to notifying the nurse in charge, which of the following actions would be **most** appropriate for the nurse to take?

① Review with June the procedures that are to occur later that day.

② Tell June that she appears troubled.

③ Remind June that she needs her sleep in preparation for the procedure.

④ Encourage June to read a magazine until she gets drowsy.

GO ON TO THE NEXT PAGE.

June has a below-the-knee amputation of her right leg as planned. Following a stay in the recovery room, June is returned to the unit.

27.   In addition to monitoring June's vital signs, the nurse should take which of the following actions **first**?

① Place her on her left side with pillows supporting the stump.

② Place her on her back with sandbags on either side of the stump.

③ Check her dressing for odor.

④ Check her dressing for bleeding.

28.   On June's second postoperative day, physical therapy is prescribed. Two days later, she refuses her breakfast and lies in bed with her face turned toward the wall. June refuses to move or to go to physical therapy. Which of the following would be best for the nurse to say **first**?

① "It's important for you to go for treatment now, June."

② "You have to stop feeling sorry for yourself if you want to get better, June."

③ "Would you rather have someone else help you, June?"

④ "Can you tell me what's bothering you, June?"

29.   During June's postoperative period, the nurse should include in the care plan a diet high in

① vitamin C and protein.

② vitamin D and carbohydrates.

③ iron and magnesium.

④ calcium and phosphorus.

30.   Which of the following developmental characteristics should the nurse take into account when planning June's care?

① Frequent mood swings.

② Difficulty expressing her feelings verbally.

③ Her need to be liked by peers.

④ Her need to be physically active.

31. June frequently puts her call light on to complain bitterly about her care. When the nurse enters her room one evening to prepare her for the night, June says, "What the hell's going on out there? Why can't I get somebody in here?" Which of the following responses should the nurse make first?

① "Everyone has to wait their turn, June. Now that I'm here, what would you like me to do?"

② "You sound terribly unhappy, June. I'll be glad to do what I can to help you."

③ "We're doing our best, June, but there are many patients here who are very ill."

④ "You must be more understanding, June. We answer your call light as quickly as we can."

32. June is experiencing phantom-limb sensation. Which of the following nursing measures should be instituted **first**?

① Exercise the stump.

② Elevate the stump.

③ Administer June's prescribed analgesic.

④ Encourage June to talk about the feeling.

Mr. George Cone and Ms. Mae Foster are elderly, widowed, and living in a residence that provides supportive services. On several occasions they have been found in each other's rooms, engaged in necking, petting, and sexual intercourse.

---

33. Mr. Cone's and Ms. Foster's sexual behavior is being discussed in a staff meeting. To arrive at a plan of action, the nurse should consider which of the following developmental needs?

① They are satisfying a physical need.

② They are acting rebelliously.

③ They are meeting an emotional need.

④ They are being exhibitionistic.

34. Mr. Cone tells the nurse that he has two full-grown sons. He frequently discusses with the nurse his parenting style and he often wonders if his sons are happy. In evaluating Mr. Cone's behavior the nurse should understand

① Mr. Cone is living in the past.

② Mr. Cone is attempting to be entertaining.

③ Mr. Cone is dealing with an unresolved conflict.

④ Mr. Cone is indulging in self-pity.

Mr. Cone has severe chest pain and is admitted to a nearby hospital.

---

35. The nurse is reading Mr. Cone's admission history. Which of the following would be **most** important to consider in reinforcing Mr. Cone's teaching?

① Drinking moderate amounts of alcoholic beverages and participating in social activities.

② Being overweight and living under persistent pressure.

③ Having irregular meal hours and living in a climate with high humidity.

④ Eating a diet high in polyunsaturated fats and getting insufficient sleep.

36. In preparing Mr. Cone for an electrocardiogram, the nurse should include which of the following information about the procedure?

① He will have nothing by mouth for 12 hours before the procedure.

② He will have no discomfort during the procedure.

③ He will be required to do mild exercise during the procedure.

③ He will have to remain flat in bed for several hours after the procedure.

37. Ms. Foster asks the nurse at the residence if she can visit Mr. Cone. Which of the following responses would be the **best** for the nurse to make?

① "I'll have to find out if Mr. Cone wants to see you."

② "I'll call Mr. Cone's unit to see if we can arrange a time."

③ "Mr. Cone will probably be back in a couple of days."

④ "Mr. Cone needs rest more than anything else."

Mr. Cone's physical condition improves and he is returned to the residence. His prescriptions include a digitalis preparation.

---

38. Which of the following statements, if made by Mr. Cone, would indicate to the nurse the need for **further** teaching?

① "I am a little thirsty today, but I should take my medicine anyway."

② "I have been urinating a little more than usual, but I should take my medicine anyway."

③ "I have been nauseated for a couple days, but I should take my medicine anyway."

④ "My pulse was 64 today, but I should take my medicine anyway."

Ms. Emma Jacobson, 43 years old, is scheduled to have a bronchoscopy. Cancer of the lung is suspected.

---

39. Following the bronchoscopy, which of the following instructions is **essential** for the nurse to give Ms. Jacobson?

① "Call me before you take a drink of anything."

② "Take deep breaths and cough every hour."

③ "Tell me when you wish to get out of bed."

④ "Avoid talking for three hours."

40. Which of the following nursing observations of Ms. Jacobson after the bronchoscopy would indicate possible complications?

① She coughs up small amounts of blood-tinged sputum.
② She complains of difficulty breathing.
③ She is very hoarse when she speaks.
④ She swallows continuously.

The results of Ms. Jacobson's diagnostic tests indicate that she has cancer of the lung. A lobectomy of her right lung is scheduled.

---

41. Ms. Jacobson expresses concern about her surgery. Which of these measures by the nurse would provide the **most** emotional support for Ms. Jacobson?

① Talking to her.
② Encouraging her family to visit.
③ Trying to cheer her up.
④ Listening to her.

42. Ms. Jacobson will have chest tubes attached to water-seal drainage following her surgery. During preoperative teaching, the nurse should emphasize that

① chest tubes allow for the removal of fluid and air.
② chest tubes make deep breathing and coughing easier.
③ chest tubes prevent rapid re-expansion of the lung.
④ chest tubes control internal hemorrhage.

Ms. Jacobson has a lobectomy of her right lung. Following a stay in the recovery room, she is brought back to her unit with a chest tube in place. Ms. Jacobson's orders include morphine sulfate q. 4h. prn, oxygen by nasal cannula, and diet as tolerated.

43. The nurse observes fluid fluctuating in Ms. Jacobson's chest tube with each respiration. Which interpretation of this observation is correct?

① Oxygen is being lost through Ms. Jacobson's chest tube.

② There is an air leak within the drainage system.

③ The apparatus is functioning properly.

④ Air is being drawn into Ms. Jacobson's chest cavity.

44. All of the following beverages are available for evening nourishment on the nursing unit. Which of the following should the nurse encourage Ms. Jacobson to drink?

① Tea with lemon.

② Apple juice.

③ Tomato juice.

④ Prune juice.

45. During the evening of the second postoperative day, Ms. Jacobson complains of pain. Which of these actions should the nurse take **first**?

① Check her chart to ascertain the time of her last pain medication.

② Take her vital signs.

③ Give her a soothing back rub and change her linen.

④ Ask her to describe her pain.

46. Ms. Jacobson is to increase her oral fluid intake, but she is reluctant to drink. Which of following nursing measures will be **most** effective in increasing her fluid intake?

① Telling her that she needs fluids to speed the healing process.

② Offering her a small glass of fluid every hour.

③ Serving her sweetened liquids between meals.

④ Keeping a pitcher of water on her bedside table.

GO ON TO THE NEXT PAGE.

Mr. Charles Walker, 69 years old, has Parkinson's disease. He is admitted to a long-term care facility. His admission orders include diet as tolerated and activity as tolerated.

47. Prior to developing Mr. Walker's nursing care plan, to which of these measures should the nurse give **priority**?

① Explain to him the roles of various nursing personnel.

② Introduce him to other long-term ambulatory clients.

③ Find out about his routines for care at home.

④ Evaluate how much he knows about his condition.

48. In planning Mr. Walker's daily care, the nurse should give the **greatest** consideration to

① completing his care in as short a time as possible.

② organizing his care so that he will feel unhurried.

③ encouraging him to assume full responsibility for his care.

④ providing long rest periods for him after each of his care activities.

49. Mr. Walker has been receiving levodopa (Larodopa). To evaluate the effectiveness of the drug, the nurse would observe for

① decreased severity of symptoms.

② remission from the disease.

③ increased resistance to infection.

④ improvement in nutritional status.

50. Mr. Walker is to have physical and occupational therapy. Which of the following measures can the nurse implement to assist Mr. Walker in his rehabilitation program?

① Giving him warm baths with massage to relax his muscles.

② Instructing him to use a cane to help him walk.

③ Showing him how to do stretching exercises to loosen his joints.

④ Encouraging him to participate in self-care activities to meet his own daily needs.

51. Mr. Walker is a journalist. One day, after trying to work on a manuscript, Mr. Walker suddenly sweeps the sheets of paper off the overbed table onto the floor. He exclaims disgustedly, "Oh, what's the use?" and starts to cry. In determining a response to the situation, which of the following should the nurse understand about Mr. Walker's behavior?

① A complete knowledge of the effects of an illness by a client insures acceptance of the illness.

② Lack of acceptance of an illness is evidenced by immature actions.

③ Clients with a chronic illness tend to seek sympathy for their condition.

④ Frustration occurs when clients can no longer be independent.

Mr. Victor Little, 82 years old, is admitted to the hospital with benign prostatic hypertrophy. He is scheduled for a transurethral prostatectomy.

---

52. Which of the following questions would be **most** appropriate for the nurse to ask when collecting data about Mr. Little's symptoms?

① "Do you have difficulty voiding?"

② "Is there a discharge from you penis?"

③ "Is there swelling in your groin?"

④ "Do you have tenderness in your scrotum?"

53. Mr. Little says to the nurse the evening before surgery, "My daughter called my minister, and he was supposed to come to see me this evening. I doubt if he will be coming now—it's 8 o'clock already." Which of the following responses would be **most** appropriate for the nurse to make initially?

① "Would you like me to check to see if your minister is still planning to come this evening, Mr. Little?"

② "Your minister keeps his word, Mr. Little. I think he'll come."

③ "Your minister may be planning to come in the morning if he can't visit you this evening."

④ "Since you feel that your minister may not come, would you like to see another minister?"

Mr. Little has a transurethral prostatectomy. When he is returned to the unit from the recovery room, he has an indwelling urethral catheter and continuous bladder irrigations with normal saline solution. An analgesic has been prescribed for him.

54. In monitoring the continuous bladder irrigation, the nurse should

① clamp the flow from the irrigating solution for the specified time, then open to allow a designated amount of solution to flush the bladder.

② infuse no more than 50 ml of irrigating solution, then apply a moderate amount of suction to withdraw the solution.

③ check to be sure that the solution out-flow corresponds to the irrigation in-flow and that the patency of the catheter is maintained.

④ warm the irrigating solution to body temperature and infuse at 100 cc per hour.

55. Mr. Little complains of pain in the bladder area, which of the following measures should the nurse take **first**?

① Find out when he received his last pain medication.

② Take his vital signs.

③ Check his urinary drainage apparatus.

④ Report his complaint to the registered nurse in charge.

56. Since Mr. Little is on continuous bladder irrigations, what color would the nurse expect his urine to be when he returns from the recovery room?

① Light pink.

② Bright red.

① Pale yellow.

④ Dark brown.

57. Mr. Little is to ambulate for the first time. Which of these actions should the nurse take **first**?

① Clamp Mr. Little's urethral catheter.

② Place an armchair along the side of Mr. Little's bed.

③ Have Mr. Little sit on the edge of the bed with his feet on a flat surface.

④ Increase the flow of the continuous bladder irrigation.

58. There is an order to remove Mr. Little's catheter. Which of the following should the nurse tell Mr. Little to expect after his catheter is removed?

① Dribbling of urine.

② Voiding large amounts of urine.

③ Foul smelling urine.

④ Light colored urine.

59. When preparing Mr. Little for discharge, which of the following instructions should the nurse reinforce?

① Refrain from walking excessively and rest as much as possible.

② Eat a low residue diet and take showers rather than baths.

③ Ignore the urge to void as long as possible and sit rather than stand to do any task.

④ Avoid straining on defecation and increase fluid intake.

Ms. Nancy Kerr, 33 years old, is admitted to the hospital with a ruptured lumbar intervertebral disc. Ms. Kerr's prescriptions include bed rest, heat applications, and meperidine hydrochloride (Demerol) prn for pain.

---

60. Before applying heat to Ms. Kerr's lower back, it is **essential** for the nurse to take which of the following actions?

① Place a plastic protective covering on the skin before applying the heat source.

② Apply a thin layer of petrolatum (Vaseline) on the skin before applying the heat source.

③ Check the temperature of the heat source.

④ Wrap the heat source in a towel.

61. Ms. Kerr requires Demerol for pain. Before giving the Demerol, it would be **most** important for the nurse to take which of the following actions?

① Check her pupillary responses.

② Count her respirations.

③ Determine her pulse deficit.

④ Assess her urinary output.

62. Which of the following techniques should the nurse utilize in assisting Ms. Kerr onto a bedpan?

① Tell her to flex her knees and raise her buttocks as the bedpan is put in place.

② Instruct her to use the overbed trapeze as a means of raising her hips so that the bedpan can be put in place.

③ Turn her onto her side, put the bedpan in place, and return her to a back-lying position on the bedpan.

④ Have her press down on the bed with her hands to raise her buttocks so that the bedpan can be put in place.

Ms. Kerr's response to medical therapy is unsatisfactory and she is scheduled for surgery.

---

63. Ms. Kerr asks the nurse if she may put makeup on before going to surgery. The nurse's **best** response would be

① "The hospital regulations state that all makeup must be removed before you go to surgery, Ms. Kerr."

② "It depends upon the amount of makeup you use, Ms. Kerr."

③ "Makeup will interfere with seeing any changes in the color of your skin during surgery, Ms. Kerr."

④ "I'll check with the nurse in charge to see if it is all right for you to put your makeup on, Ms. Kerr."

Ms. Kerr has a laminectomy performed under general anesthesia. After several hours in the recovery room, Ms. Kerr is returned to her unit.

---

64. Ms. Kerr's blood pressure has been stable at 130/80, and her pulse rate has been 80. Which of the following vital signs would indicate to the nurse the development of shock?

① Blood pressure 100/60; pulse 120.

② Blood pressure 120/80; pulse 74.

③ Blood pressure 140/100; pulse 100.

④ Blood pressure 150/90; pulse 60.

65. Ms. Kerr is ambulatory. She complains of a sore area in her left calf. Which of the following actions by the nurse would be **most** appropriate?

① Instruct Ms. Kerr to remain in bed and then report the symptom to the nurse in charge.

② Massage Ms. Kerr's left leg gently and then assess her pedal pulse.

③ Have Ms. Kerr ambulate and then question her about the effect of the activity on her left leg.

④ Tell Ms. Kerr to move her left leg and then palpate it for other areas of soreness.

Mr. Frank Anderman, 85 years old, has been in a long-term care facility for 10 months. He is confused at times and has generalized arteriosclerosis.

---

66. The nurse would expect Mr. Anderman to be most confused and disoriented during which of the following times?

① Upon arising in the morning.

② When ambulating during the day.

③ When sitting alone in the afternoon.

④ Upon awakening during the night.

67. Mr. Anderman may have a diet as tolerated. In collecting data about his nutritional needs the nurse should be **most** concerned about his

① age.

② ability to chew.

③ activity level.

④ food preferences.

68. In planning Mr. Anderman's nutritional requirements the nurse should consider Mr. Anderman has a decreased need for

① vitamin B complex.

② calcium.

③ protein.

④ calories.

69. When the nurse is preparing Mr. Anderman for sleep, he says, "I wake up at night because my feet get so cold. How can I keep them warm?" Which of the following actions would be **best** for the nurse to take?

① Rub his feet briskly to improve the circulation.

② Place a light blanket over his feet.

③ Place his feet on a covered hot-water bottle.

④ Put a covered heating pad on his feet, with the dial turned to the lowest setting.

Ms. Pamela Evan, 54 years old, is admitted to the hospital for a subtotal gastrectomy. Her preoperative orders include a cleansing enema.

---

70. Ms. Evan is to receive an enema of 1,000 ml. of solution. After receiving 100 ml. of the solution, Ms. Evan says to the nurse, "I can't hold any more. It's going to come out!" Which of these actions would it be most appropriate for the nurse to take **first**?

① Remove the rectal tube, place Ms. Evan on the bedpan, and then attempt to give the remainder of the fluid later if she still needs it.

② Clamp the tubing, instruct Ms. Evan to take several deep breaths, and then wait a minute or two before releasing the clamp.

③ Inform Ms. Evan that additional fluid must be instilled, lower the fluid container slightly, and continue the procedure.

④ Discontinue the procedure, place Ms. Evan on the bedpan, and then report the problem to the nurse in charge.

71. In planning Ms. Evan's preoperative care, the nurse should

① give the preoperative medication prior to morning care to allow for observation of Ms. Evan's reaction to the medication.

② give the preoperative medication prior to morning care to promote optimal relaxation in Ms. Evan.

③ complete Ms. Evan's morning care prior to giving her preoperative medication to prevent having to disturb her.

④ complete Ms. Evan's morning care prior to giving her preoperative medication because the medication will act rapidly in a person of her age.

72. After Ms. Evan is transferred from the stretcher to her bed, the nurse takes her vital signs. Which of the following actions should the nurse take **next**?

① Have Ms. Evan deep breathe.

② Determine Ms. Evan's need for medication to relieve pain.

③ Check Ms. Evan's level of consciousness.

④ Inspect Ms. Evan's dressing.

73. While Ms. Evan has the nasogastric tube in place, her plan of care includes frequent mouth care for the purpose of

① maintaining her ability to swallow.

② preventing her from loosing her gag reflex.

③ keeping the oral mucous membrane moist.

④ stimulating peristalsis.

74. During the early postoperative period, the nurse encourages Ms. Evan to move her lower extremities frequently in order to prevent

① pressure sores.

② abdominal distention.

③ muscle atrophy.

④ venous stasis.

75. On the evening prior to surgery, the nurse is reinforcing the need for Ms. Turner to cough and deep breathe. She says, "Stop treating me like a child. I wouldn't be here now if I hadn't learned to breathe a long time ago." Which of the following responses would be **most** appropriate for the nurse to make?

① "Do you know the reason for doing this?"

② "Do you feel I'm talking down to you?"

③ "You're overreacting."

④ "No one else has had that complaint."

76. On the morning of her surgery, Ms. Turner has a nasogastric tube inserted. The nurse should explain that the purpose of this procedure is to

① remove gas and fluids from the stomach.

② promote peristalsis in the large intestine.

③ prevent accumulation of fecal matter in the large intestine.

④ provide a means of administering nourishment postoperatively.

77. In Ms. Turner's early postoperative care, it would be most important for the nurse to take measures to

① improve her respiratory function.

② increase her nutritional intake.

③ establish a routine pattern for urine elimination.

④ promote expulsion of flatus.

78. When changing Ms. Turner's ileostomy bag, it is **most** important for the nurse to take which of the following measures?

① Refrain from showing distaste.

② Maintain strict surgical asepsis.

③ Explain the details of the procedures.

④ Wipe the stoma with a mild antiseptic.

79. Arrangements are made for Ms. Turner to be visited by a woman who has adjusted well to her ileostomy. Which of the following actions by the nurse would be **most** helpful in promoting the effectiveness of the visit?

① Remain in the room while the session is in progress.

② Return to the room periodically to answer any questions that may arise.

③ Provide a quiet, private setting for the visit.

④ Maintain a detached manner until the visit is over.

80. On several occasions, Ms. Turner is observed picking at the food on her tray and eating very little. When questioned by the nurse, Ms. Turner says that she doesn't feel like eating. Which of the following actions by the nurse would be **most** appropriate?

① Ask Ms. Turner if she would like her husband to bring in food from home.

② Explain to Ms. Turner the importance of good nutrition to her recovery.

③ Explain to Ms. Turner that her refusal to eat will have to be reported to the physician.

④ Ask Ms. Turner if she likes the meals she has been served.

Mr. Spencer Otto, 22 years old, is brought to the emergency room following a motorcycle accident. He has a head injury and is semicomatose.

---

81. When Mr. Otto arrives in the emergency room, the **initial** action that should be taken by the nurse is to

① check his vital signs.

② assess the extent of his injury.

③ determine the patency of his airway.

④ institute measures to prevent infection.

82. In preparation for the lumber puncture, the nurse should place Mr. Otto in which of the following positions?

① Lateral decubitus with knees to abdomen and neck flexed.

② Supine with a trochanter roll parallel to the thighs and arms extended.

③ Prone with head turned to one side and the legs slightly elevated.

④ Fowler's with a pillow under the lower back and feet abducted.

83. Which of the following nursing interventions is **most** important during Mr. Otto's lumbar puncture?

① Explain to the client the steps of the procedure as they occur.

② Help the client to remain motionless.

③ Prepare the labels for the fluid specimens.

④ Apply pressure to the insertion site as the needle is being removed.

84. One morning when the nurse enters Mr. Otto's room he starts to have a seizure. After assuring Mr. Otto's safety, which of the following actions should the nurse take **next**?

① Suction his oropharynx.

② Restrain his extremities.

③ Help him to turn onto his abdomen after the seizure.

④ Observe what occurs during the seizure.

85. Which of the following observations by the nurse would indicate increased intracranial pressure?

① Oliguria.

② Pallor.

③ Lethargy.

④ Hypothermia.

Mrs. Ada Johnson, 89 years old, is admitted to an extended care facility. She has Alzheimer's disease, has been bedridden for two years, and has contractures of her extremities.

86.   Ms. Johnson grabs at the nurse. Which of the following actions would be **most** appropriate for the nurse to take?

① Apply a chest restraint and tell Ms. Johnson that this is for her safety.

② Reprimand Ms. Johnson and remind her that this behavior is harmful.

③ Remove Ms. Johnson's hands and tell her that this behavior makes it difficult to perform nursing care.

④ Move away from Ms. Johnson's reach and leave the room until she becomes calmer.

87.   Because of Ms. Johnson's agitation, which of the following measures would be **best** for the nurse to include in Ms. Johnson's plan of care?

① Keep her room dimly lit, the side rails up, and stimulation at a minimum.

② Place her in a geri-chair at the nurses' station and give her small simple tasks which are repetitious in nature.

③ Apply restraints and monitor her hourly.

④ Move her close to the nurses station, turn on a radio to soothing music, and check her frequently.

88.   In order to prevent further contractures, which of the following measures should the nurse implement for Ms. Johnson?

① Place her in a warm whirlpool bath daily.

② Exercise her joints to the limit of her range of motion qid.

③ Turn her from side to side every two hours.

④ Support the contracted joints on pillows at all times.

Mr. Jack Trenton, 70 years old, resides in an extended care facility. He was recently found in bed, restless and disoriented, complaining of shortness of breath. His temperature was 39.4°C (103°F). He is diagnosed as having pneumonia. Antibiotics and bronchodilators are prescribed.

89. Because Mr. Trenton is restless and confused, which of the following methods would be the **best** for the nurse to use in taking his vital signs?

① Take an apical pulse and a rectal temperature.

② Take a radial pulse and an oral temperature.

③ Take a femoral pulse and an axillary temperature.

④ Take a carotid pulse and an axillary temperature.

90. When Mr. Trenton is less restless and confused, the physician orders postural drainage bid. The **best** time for the nurse to perform postural drainage is

① when Mr. Trenton arises and 1 hour before he retires.

② after Mr. Trenton has had breakfast and before supper.

③ 60 minutes before Mr. Trenton's lunch and after his antibiotics are administered.

④ 30 minutes before Mr. Trenton's morning care and after his bronchodilators are administered.

91. Mr. Trenton uses a walker to ambulate. In assisting him with the walker, it would be best for the nurse to

① walk directly behind him.

② walk in front of him, guiding the walker.

③ walk closely behind and slightly to the side of him.

④ walk beside him.

92.   Which of the following statements made by Ms. Chapman would indicate to the nurse that she is adapting to a reduced energy level?

① "I'm too tired to do much anymore. I don't think I can even put away my mail."

② "Can you take me to the dining room in a wheelchair? I'm too tired to walk."

③ "I'm going to take a nap. Maybe I'll exercise later."

④ "Even though I'm tired, I can go down to play bingo."

93.   Ms. Chapman becomes upset each time she is taken to the bathing room to use the whirlpool tub. Which of the following nursing measures should be implemented to reduce her anxiety?

① Arrange to have her bathe last.

② Demonstrate the equipment so she feels comfortable using it.

③ Suggest she take bed baths.

④ Stay with her during the procedure to assist her as needed.

94.   Ms. Chapman experiences stress incontinence. Which of the following measures would be **best** for the nurse to take in helping Ms. Chapman adapt to this problem?

① Inform her that this is due to an infection and will only be temporary.

② Instruct her in muscle-strengthening exercises.

③ Provide frequent bathing and protection for her garments.

④ Assist her with ordering an incontinence brief.

95. In evaluating the sleep patterns of an elderly client, the nurse should understand that the elderly

① have no fundamental changes in sleep patterns.

② sleep soundly throughout the night.

③ arouse more frequently during the night.

④ require less sleep as they grow older.

96. An elderly client has a left cataract extraction as an out-patient. Which of the following statements by the client would indicate to the nurse the need for **further** teaching?

① "Sleeping on my back is OK."

② "I can take Tylenol for discomfort."

③ "Feeling nauseous is normal after surgery."

④ "If I get constipated, I should call the doctor."

97. To assist in reducing a client's body temperature, the nurse should place cool, moist packs on the

① groin and axillae.

② neck and feet.

③ chest and back.

④ hands and forehead.

98. The nurse, assisting with a pelvic examination, requests that the patient empty her bladder prior to the procedure. The client wants to know why this is necessary. Which of the following would be the **best** response by the nurse?

① "It prevents possible rupture of a distended bladder."

② "It assists in visualization of the vaginal canal."

③ "It aids in assessment of the pelvic organs."

④ "It helps you to relax during the procedure."

99. An alcoholic client is admitted to the hospital. Which of the following would the nurse observe as early signs of delirium tremens?

① Muscle rigidity and tension.

② Agitation and anger.

③ Restlessness and confusion.

④ Abdominal distention and lethargy.

100. A client is on a high-protein, high-calorie diet. Which of the following menus should the nurse encourage the client to select?

① Bacon, lettuce, and tomato sandwich, fruited gelatin dessert with whipped topping, and a cola.

② Roast beef sandwich, mashed potatoes with gravy, green beans, chocolate pudding, and fruit punch.

③ Ground beef patty, cucumber salad, cooked carrots, apple, and orange juice.

④ Macaroni with tomato sauce, spinach, pear, and milk.

101. A child is in the acute stage of rheumatic fever. In planning this child's care, the nurse should maximize the child's

① rest.

② fluids.

③ exercise.

④ social interaction.

102. In reinforcing teaching for a diabetic client, the nurse should be certain that the client has which of the following understandings about the management of insulin-dependent diabetes mellitus?

① Urine which is glucose-free is the best indicator of diabetes mellitus under control.

② Symptoms of any illness necessitates immediate notification of the physician.

③ Diabetes mellitus can be cured if measures prescribed by the physician are followed.

④ Self-regulation of medication indicates good management of the disease process.

103. In monitoring a client's condition after a dilatation and curettage (D and C), which of the following would be **most** important for the nurse to observe?

① Temperature elevation.

② Vaginal bleeding.

③ Bladder distention.

④ Voluntary leg movements.

104. A client asks the nurse why bathing with a povidone-iodine solution (Betadine) must be done prior to surgery. The nurse's reply is based on the understanding that this procedure is done to

① sterilize the skin.

② improve circulation to the surgical area.

③ avoid contamination of the operating room.

④ reduce the possibility of infection.

105. A client is receiving oxygen therapy by mask. Which of the following measures should the nurse include in the plan of care?

① Taking the temperature rectally.

② Giving a complete bed bath.

③ Urging additional fluids.

④ Assisting with coughing and deep breathing exercises.

106. A client with constipation is to be given both an oil retention enema and a cleansing enema. Which of the following procedures should the nurse undertake to produce the **best** results?

① The cleansing enema is given before the oil retention enema.

② The cleansing enema is given immediately after the oil retention enema.

③ The oil retention enema is given first and allowed to remain in the bowel for a period of time before the cleansing enema is given.

④ The solutions for the oil retention enema and the cleansing enema are thoroughly mixed and given together at the same time.

107. A client has had a resection of her right lung. She has a chest tube and is receiving oxygen. In addition to administering her prescribed analgesic, which of the following actions should the nurse take that would **best** assist the client to cough and deep breathe?

① Splinting the chest with a pillow.

② Elevating the head of the bed.

③ Clamping the chest tube.

④ Removing the oxygen temporarily.

108. A client has a freshly applied plaster cast on the right leg. Which of the following measures should the nurse take?

① Place a waterproof protection around the cast.

② Use a heat lamp to reduce the cast's drying time.

③ Smooth rough edges of the cast by feathering.

④ Elevate the casted right leg on pillows.

109. A client is receiving aminophylline (Theophylline) for pulmonary emphysema which has been complicated by an upper respiratory infection. To evaluate the effectiveness of the drug, the nurse should monitor the

① amount and color of secretions.

② rate and rhythm of respirations.

③ pattern of temperature elevations.

④ expansion of the chest cavity.

110. To facilitate breathing in a client with respiratory distress, the nurse should place the client in which of the following positions?

① Supine.

② Trendelenburg.

③ Fowler's.

④ Sims'.

111. A client is being prepared for an amniocentesis. Prior to the procedure the nurse should instruct the client to

① refrain from eating.

② take an enema.

③ empty her bladder.

④ scrub her abdomen.

112. When assessing a client three hours after a normal vaginal delivery, the following observations are noted: fundus is firm, 2 fingerbreadths above the umbilicus, and displaced to the left of the midline. Based on these observations, which of the following actions would be **most** appropriate for the nurse to take?

① Massage the fundus.

② Notify the nurse in charge.

③ Instruct the client to void.

④ Record the information on the client's chart.

113. A diabetic client has been taught how to give her own insulin. Which of the following statements would indicate to the nurse the client understands the teaching?

① "I will limit contact with others to avoid infections."

② "I will refrigerate the insulin bottle I am using."

③ "I should not take my insulin if I am vomiting."

④ "I can continue my exercise classes three times a week."

114. Phototherapy is instituted because a newborn has jaundice. Which of the following precautions should the nurse institute during the therapy?

① Withhold the infant's feedings.

② Shield the infant's eyes.

③ Monitor the infant's temperature every hour.

④ Cover the infant's trunk.

115. A client is receiving a thiazide diuretic. Which of the following foods should the nurse encourage the client to include in his diet?

① Milk.

② Apricots.

③ Pork.

④ Beets.

116. A client has vascular occlusion of the left leg. Which of the following approaches should the nurse include in her assessment?

① Comparing the pulses in the lower extremities.

② Comparing the temperature of the lower extremities.

③ Noting the pulse in the left leg.

④ Noting the temperature of the left leg.

117. A client has been taught crutch walking. Which of the following observations by the nurse would indicate a need for **further** instructions?

① The client is wearing tennis shoes.

② The client is bearing weight on the axillae.

③ The client advances the affected leg with the crutches.

④ The client places the crutches 8 to 10 inches out in front with each step.

118. A client has severe renal impairment. Which of the following nutrients would the nurse expect to be restricted in the diet?

① Cholesterol.

② Carbohydrates.

③ Fats.

④ Proteins.

119. A client undergoes cystoscopic examination under local anesthesia. Following the procedure, the nurse should be **most** concerned about which of the following complaints?

① Leg cramps.

② Nausea.

③ Headache.

④ Low abdominal discomfort.

120. A client has a chest tube attached to water-seal drainage. Which of the following nursing measures is **most** important in preventing respiratory complications?

① Securing the tubing above the level of the incision.

② Reinforcing the dressing over the insertion site.

③ Sealing the vent on the suction control chamber of the water-seal drainage system.

④ Keeping the water-seal drainage system near floor level.

The National Council Licensure Examination for Practical Nurses

PART II

**You will be allowed 2 hours
to complete this part of the examination.**

Please begin.

Ms. Ann Lasher, 20 years old, attends the antepartal clinic. The physician examines Ms. Lasher and finds her to be about 12 weeks pregnant.

121. Ms. Lasher states that she never drinks milk. The nurse asks if she is allergic to milk. Ms. Lasher answers, "No, I just don't like the taste of it." Which of the following responses by the nurse would be **best**?

① "What foods do you like that contain milk?"

② "Do you understand why milk is important for the development of your baby?"

③ "Substitute 1 whole egg for every glass of milk that you omit from your diet."

④ "Talk with your physician about taking calcium tablets as a substitute for milk."

122. Ms. Lasher states that she works out 3 or 4 times a week and asks how much exercise she can safely do while she is pregnant. Which of the following responses by the nurse would be **best**?

① "Activities that require stretching and bending should be avoided."

② "Usual activities should be continued in moderation."

③ "Emphasis should be given to active participation in outdoor activities."

④ "Each new activity should be preceded by a short period of rest."

123. When Baby Girl Lasher is brought to Ms. Lasher for the first breast-feeding, Ms. Lasher asks the nurse, "How much of the nipple should the baby be given?" Which of these following replies would be **best** for the nurse to give Ms. Lasher?

① "The baby should have the nipple and some of the dark area around the nipple well into her mouth."

② "Since she's had some water from a bottle in the nursery, she has already learned the amount of nipple she needs to adequately nurse."

③ "Babies' mouths are of different sizes, and the baby will take the correct amount of nipple for her."

④ "Babies nurse best when only the nipple is in the mouth."

124. On Ms. Lasher's second postpartum day, the nurse finds Ms. Lasher crying. When asked what seems to be wrong, Ms. Lasher says, "I really don't know. I have so much to be grateful for—a healthy baby, a good husband—I really should be happy." Which of the following actions by the nurse would demonstrate the **best** judgment in this situation?

① Provide privacy for Ms. Lasher.

② Ask Ms. Lasher if her relationship with her husband will permit her to discuss her feelings with him.

③ Explain to Ms. Lasher that her reaction is an unusual one.

④ Remain with Ms. Lasher for a while.

125. Because Ms. Lasher is breast-feeding her baby, which of the following changes in her diet should the nurse reinforce?

① Decrease roughage and increase carbohydrates.

② Decrease sodium and increase iron.

③ Increase calcium and protein.

④ Increase fats and carbohydrates.

126.   While collecting data from Ms. Quinn, the nurse would expect Ms. Quinn to complain of

① loss of appetite and abnormal pigmentation.

② insomnia and palpitations.

③ polyuria and excessive thirst.

④ diaphoresis and disorientation.

127.   The physician has ordered a protein-bound iodine (PBI), a radioactive iodine uptake, and a T-3 uptake test. Which of the following instructions should the nurse give in preparing Ms. Quinn for these diagnostic measures?

① Food and fluids are restricted prior to the procedures.

② Proper imaging of the thyroid during the tests requires restricting movement.

③ The tests may take some time because the dyes injected travel slowly to the thyroid.

④ Ingestion of iodine is restricted prior to the tests.

128.   The medical diagnosis of hyperthyroidism is confirmed. The nursing diagnosis of altered nutrition: less than body requirements is established. Which of the following diets should the nurse encourage Ms. Quinn to eat?

① High-fluid, high-fiber diet.

② High-calorie with vitamin and carbohydrate supplements.

③ Low-carbohydrate, high-protein diet.

④ Low-fat with vitamin and calcium supplements.

129.   The physician prescribes a liquid oral iodine solution prior to scheduling Ms. Quinn for thyroid surgery. In reinforcing instructions, which of the following statements by Ms. Quinn would indicate to the nurse that Ms. Quinn understands the instructions?

① "The drug must be taken on an empty stomach."

② "The drug should be taken prior to noon."

③ "The drug should be diluted and taken through a straw."

④ "The drug will cause a flushed feeling when ingested."

130. When Ms. Quinn is admitted to the hospital for her thyroidectomy, a nursing diagnosis of ineffective thermoregulation is established. In planning her care the nurse should

① keep the room as cool as possible.
② provide extra blankets at night.
③ encourage frequent bathing.
④ monitor her vital signs frequently.

131. Ms. Quinn has a subtotal thyroidectomy. When she has completely reacted from anesthesia and her vital signs are stable, which of the following positions should the nurse place her in?

① Prone.
② Supported Fowler's.
③ Sims'.
④ Supine.

Steve Holmes, 8 years old, has sickle cell anemia. He is admitted to the hospital in sickle cell crisis.

---

132. Steve is complaining of pain in his legs and abdomen. Steve's mother is concerned and asks the nurse what causes the pain. Which of the following responses would be **best** for the nurse to make?

① "The pain is caused by bleeding into the cellular spaces."
② "The pain is caused by clumping of red blood cells."
③ "The pain is caused by a generalized infection."
④ "The pain is caused by a shift of intestinal fluid."

133. Steve is very quiet and lies facing the wall much of the time. Which of the following measures would be **best** for the nurse to include in Steve's nursing care plan?

① Spend time with Steve other than when giving him physical care.
② Provide Steve with an opportunity to talk with an older child who also has sickle cell anemia.
③ Assure Steve at frequent intervals that he is improving.
④ Remind Steve that being upset might make his condition worse.

134. Which of the following statements, if made by Ms. Holmes, would indicate to the nurse that Ms. Holmes understands sickle cell anemia?

① "Sickle cell anemia can be controlled if the disease is diagnosed at birth."

② "Sickle cell anemia is a disease characterized by periods of crisis throughout life."

③ "If a child with sickle cell anemia is in remission for two years, the disease is considered arrested."

④ "When a child with sickle cell anemia reaches puberty, crises will no longer occur."

135. In planning Steve's play activities, which of the following should the nurse consider?

① Eight-year-olds need to have highly structured activities.

② Eight-year-olds prefer being with children of the opposite sex.

③ Eight-year-olds like to be involved with a group of children their own age.

④ Eight-year-olds usually include an imaginary playmate in their activities.

Steve's condition improves, and plans are made with Ms. Holmes for his discharge.

---

136. Ms. Holmes says to the nurse, "We're planning to go camping at a lake for the entire summer. It's about 400 from here." Which of the following statements would be **most** appropriate for the nurse to make to Ms. Holmes?

① "Be sure that Steve is not exposed to the sun."

② "Plan to drive for only short periods at a time so that Steve will have a chance to exercise his legs."

③ "Limit Steve's fluids while traveling to help prevent him from being carsick."

④ "Ask your physician about the medical facilities that are available where you are going."

137. In monitoring Harry for antibiotic hypersensitivity, which of the following should the nurse observe for?

① Anorexia.

② Urticaria.

③ Constipation.

④ Hypertension.

138. In the early postoperative period, which of the following should the nurse consider in planning Harry's pain management?

① Analgesia is necessary and is safe if the dosage is calculated for the individual child.

② Potential drug addiction should be a concern in the care of an acutely ill child.

③ Since children are active earlier in the postoperative period than adults, they will need little or no analgesia.

④ Children have a higher tolerance for pain than do adults and therefore need smaller doses of drugs.

139. In planning Harry's care, which of the following should the nurse consider?

① Twelve-year-olds reject new routines.

② Twelve-year-olds are shy when meeting new people.

③ Twelve-year-olds are anxious when separated from parents.

④ Twelve-year-olds need privacy.

Ms. Toni Hale, 33 years old, is seen in the clinic with acute pyelonephritis. Ms. Hale is to be on bed rest and have fluids ad lib. A urine specimen for culture and sensitivity is ordered.

140.   Ms. Hale asks the nurse why she has to stay in bed. Which of the following would be the **best** response by the nurse?

① "To prevent respiratory infection by reducing your contact with other people."

② "To insure safety while you have toxins in your bloodstream."

③ "To assist your body's defenses in combating infection."

④ "To control ascending urinary infection by maintaining a horizontal position."

141.   To obtain a urine specimen for culture and sensitivity from Ms. Hale, which of these actions by the nurse is **essential**?

① Encourage her to drink fluids before the urine is collected.

② Place a preservative in the receptacle in which her urine is to be collected.

③ Collect the first urine that she voids in the morning.

④ Use aseptic technique in collecting her urine.

142.   Ms. Hale's urine sample for culture and sensitivity is cloudy and contains threads of mucous and blood. Which of the following actions should be taken by the nurse?

① Record and report the observations.

② Obtain a different urine specimen for the test.

② Strain the urine before sending it to the lab.

④ Notify the lab of the contaminated specimen.

143. Ms. Stone has been advised by the physician to increase her intake of iron. Which of the following sandwiches, if selected by Ms. Stone, would indicate to the nurse that Ms. Stone understands the need for increased dietary iron?

① Egg salad.

② Peanut butter.

③ Cream cheese and jelly.

④ Lettuce and tomato.

144. While attending the clinic during her eighth month, Ms. Stone says to the nurse, "Sometimes I think about what would happen if I died during childbirth." Which of the following responses by the nurse would be **best**?

① "These thoughts are common at your stage of pregnancy."

② "Maternal deaths are extremely rare."

③ "What has prompted these feelings in you?"

④ "Have you discussed these feelings with your husband?"

At term, Ms. Stone is admitted to the hospital in active labor which progresses normally. She delivers a boy. Ms. Stone is transferred to the postpartum unit.

145. A few hours after Ms. Stone's delivery, the nurse notes that Ms. Stone has saturated two perineal pads with blood within a 20-minute period. Which of the following actions should the nurse take **first**?

① Check the consistency of Ms. Stone's uterine fundus.

② Encourage Ms. Stone to void.

③ Take Ms. Stone's blood pressure.

④ Notify the nurse in charge.

GO ON TO THE NEXT PAGE.

146. Ms. Stone says to the nurse, "I guess I really need some help. I don't want any more children. Three are enough." Which of the following approaches by the nurse should be taken **first**?

① Find out what Ms. Stone knows about the availability of family planning services.

② Ask Ms. Stone if her husband is interested in birth control.

③ Discuss with Ms. Stone the effectiveness of various contraceptive methods.

④ Commend Ms. Stone for her determination to limit her family size.

Ms. Liane Wilson, 37 years old, has six children, aged 1, 2, 3, 5, 7, and 9 years. Ms. Wilson is visiting the physician because she has not menstruated for several months.

---

147. In the waiting room, Ms. Wilson says to another client, "Here I am again. I kind of hope that I'm not pregnant." When the nurse is helping Ms. Wilson prepare for her examination, the nurse says to Ms. Wilson, "I overheard your comments to the other patient in the waiting room." Which of the following statements by the nurse would be **most** appropriate to follow this initial comment?

① "You may feel negative about another pregnancy now, but these feelings are bound to change."

② "It's healthy to express your feelings. Let's talk about them."

③ "You ought to discuss these feelings with the doctor, since they may affect the outcome of your pregnancy."

④ "The doctor may advise you to seek professional counseling. Such feelings often precede emotional problems in the postpartum period."

148. The physician confirms that Ms. Wilson is about 12 weeks pregnant. As she is leaving the physician's office, Ms. Wilson says to the nurse, "The doctor wants me to keep all of my appointments and follow his directions carefully. After 6 babies I can take care of myself." Which of the following responses by the nurse would be **best**?

① "You are at risk of premature labor because you are extremely active and over 35 years of age."
② "Your baby is prone to lack of oxygen because of your age."
③ "Your baby is especially susceptible to infections because you are around young children."
④ "You have a higher incidence of complications because you have had several previous pregnancies and are over 35 years of age."

At term Ms. Wilson is admitted to the hospital and delivers a 9-lb, 4-oz (4,196-gm) boy. Ms. Wilson is planning to breast-feed her baby.

---

149. Ms. Wilson expresses concern about her ability to supply the baby with enough milk because of his large size. Which of the following responses by the nurse would be **best**?

① "Supplemental feedings can be added for babies who weigh more than 9 pounds."
② "Eight to ten glasses of fluid per day will insure an adequate milk supply."
③ "Milk production is enhanced by avoiding certain foods, alcohol, and smoking."
④ "The more the baby sucks, the more milk the breasts will produce to meet the baby's needs."

150. The nurse is reinforcing teaching regarding oral contraceptives. Which of the following statements, if made by Ms. Wilson, would indicate to the nurse Ms. Wilson understands the teaching?

① "They are quite effective in women whose menstrual cycle is regular."
② "They vary in effectiveness according to the woman's age."
③ "They are very effective when taken exactly as prescribed."
④ "They are highly effective only if used in conjunction with a birth control device such as a diaphragm."

151. Which of the following instructions regarding Linda's care is it **most** important for the nurse to reinforce for Ms. Malone?

① Bathe Linda daily with a mild soap.

② Keep Linda's nails cut short.

③ Use only long-sleeved clothing for Linda.

④ Have the other children in the family avoid contact with Linda.

152. In collecting data about Linda, the nurse would expect Linda to

① hold her bottle during a feeding.

② smile in response to being talked to.

③ turn from her back to her abdomen.

④ cry when a stranger approaches.

153. Linda is wearing elbow restraints. At which of these times would it be appropriate for the nurse to remove Linda's restraints?

① When Linda is being held.

② When Linda is sleeping.

③ When Linda is being transported in a carriage.

④ When Linda is having her dressing changed.

154. Linda is receiving an antihistamine. In evaluating the outcome of this medication, the nurse should expect

① enhanced healing of the lesions.

② reduced itching of the lesions.

③ limited spread of the lesions.

④ prevented infection of the lesions.

155. In collecting data on admission, which objective sign observed by the nurse would be indicative of an inguinal hernia?

① Protrusion of the umbilicus.

② Visible peristalsis.

③ A mass in the groin.

④ Abdominal distention.

156. Bobby arrives at the hospital clutching a rather soiled, ragged blanket. When his mother attempts to remove the blanket to take it home, Bobby cries and holds on to it. Which of the following comments by the nurse would indicate the **best** understanding of Bobby's needs?

① ''It looks as if that's Bobby's favorite blanket. It's all right for him to keep it with him.''

① ''Let's wait until Bobby is involved in an activity, then I'll take the blanket and give it to you next time you come.''

③ ''I'll get Bobby another blanket. Then he won't mind giving up this one.''

④ ''Tell Bobby that you only want to take the blanket to wash it and that you'll bring it back next time you come.''

157. Bobby is to have a venipuncture to obtain a blood specimen. When the physician is ready to take Bobby's blood, which of the following approaches by the nurse would be **best**?

① Tell Bobby which arm to extend to the physician.

② Hold Bobby's arm in position for the physician.

③ Show Bobby how to squeeze his fist tight while the needle is being inserted.

④ Have Bobby cover his eyes with one hand while the specimen is being withdrawn.

GO ON TO THE NEXT PAGE.

158. Ms. Tate tells the nurse that she has to leave because she has a 6-month-old baby at home. Ms. Tate says, "Bobby has never been away from home without me and I think he's going to be very upset." Which of the following responses would be **best** for the nurse to make?

① "Maybe if you promise to bring him his favorite toy when you return, he won't cry so much."

② "If we hear Bobby crying, we will send someone in to care for him."

③ "I'll stay here with Bobby and try to comfort him."

④ "Most children only cry for a little while after their mothers leave."

Bobby is scheduled for surgery and is to have nothing by mouth.

---

159. While Bobby can have nothing by mouth, he is unhappy and cries for something to drink. Which of the following measures would it be appropriate for the nurse to include in his care plan?

① Take Bobby for a walk.

② Give Bobby ice chips to suck.

③ Have Bobby use a pleasant-flavored mouthwash.

④ Explain to Bobby why he cannot have fluids.

Bobby has surgery. He is to be discharged the next day.

---

160. Ms. Tate tells the nurse that the Bobby does not drink enough milk. Which of the following foods could the nurse suggest as a substitute for milk?

① Citrus fruit juices.

② Cream.

③ Cheese.

④ Root vegetables.

161. The nurse is unable to count Anna's respirations accurately because she is restless and crying. Which of the following actions by the nurse would be **best**?

① Ask another staff member to count Anna's respirations.

② Record an approximate respiratory rate.

③ Postpone taking Anna's respirations until she becomes quiet.

④ Average her respirations per minute after taking them for three minutes.

162. The evening after Anna's admission, Ms. Garcia arrives to visit Anna. Ms. Garcia says to the nurse, "I just put my hand in the tent. Anna's clothing is damp." In addition to changing Anna's clothing, which of the following actions should the nurse take in response to Ms. Garcia's comment?

① Report Ms. Garcia's observation to the nurse in charge.

② Encourage Anna to drink fluids to replace those she is losing.

③ Take Anna's temperature to compare it with her previous temperature.

④ Explain the function of the humidity to Ms. Garcia.

163. Before returning Anna to the croup tent, the nurse should take which of the following actions?

① Close the tent and turn on the oxygen flow meter.

② Wipe the inside of the canopy with a disinfectant solution.

③ Hold Anna and explain why she has to be returned to the croup tent.

④ Assist Anna in doing deep-breathing exercises.

Anna's condition has improved. She is ambulatory and ready for discharge.

164. Anna is in the playroom. Which of these behaviors would the nurse observe in a typical 2-year-old child?

① Playing a simple board game with another child of the same age.

② Sitting quietly with a group of children while listening to a story.

③ Coloring within the lines of drawings in a coloring book, using jumbo-size crayons.

④ Engaging in activities near other children but not with them.

Ms. Ida Young, 65 years old, complains of coldness, numbness, and tingling sensations in her lower extremities. There is an area of ulceration on her left ankle. Ms. Young is admitted to the hospital with peripheral vascular disease and insulin-dependent diabetes mellitus. Her admission orders include warm, moist packs to the ulcer.

165. Which of the following items should the nurse add to Ms. Young's bed?

① Bed board.

② Bed cradle.

③ Shock blocks.

④ Trapeze bar.

166. In applying the warm, moist packs to Ms. Young's ankle, the nurse should use aseptic technique for which of the following purposes?

① To destroy bacteria on the skin.

② To inhibit the growth of pathogens.

③ To prevent the introduction of additional microorganisms.

④ To minimize the risk of spreading infection to others.

167.　Ms. Young's diabetes mellitus has not been controlled, the nurse should observe Ms. Young for which of the following symptoms?

① Anorexia and constipation.

② Tremors and irritability.

③ Polydipsia and polyuria.

④ Weight gain and diaphoresis.

The physician prescribes a 1,500-calorie diabetic diet and 30 units of isophane (NPH) insulin daily for Ms. Young.

168.　Ms. Young is to have a midafternoon snack of milk and crackers. Ms. Young asks the nurse why she has to have this snack. Which of the following responses by the nurse would be **best**?

① "It will improve your nutrition."

② "It improves your carbohydrate metabolism."

③ "It prevents an insulin reaction."

④ "It prevents diabetic coma."

169.　While the nurse is administering the insulin injection, Ms. Young asks, "Why can't you give me a pill?" Which of the following responses by the nurse would be **best**?

① "Oral drugs cannot be used to treat your type of diabetes."

② "Oral drugs used to treat diabetes act less rapidly than insulin by injection."

③ "An oral drug is a natural product whereas insulin for injection is a synthetic product."

④ "Ask your doctor if you can switch from insulin injections to an oral drug."

170.　One day the nurse enters the room just as Ms. Young is lighting a cigarette. Ms. Young says, "My doctor has advised me to stop smoking. Why is that?" Which of the following responses by the nurse would be **best**?

① "Smoking cigarettes produces constriction of blood vessels."

② "Smoking causes cancer."

③ "Smoking irritates your lungs."

④ "Smoking causes hardening of the arteries."

GO ON TO THE NEXT PAGE.

171. In caring for Ms. Young, the nurse should include which of the following in Ms. Young's foot care program?

① Soak her feet daily in water containing magnesium sulfate (Epsom salt).

② Cut her toenails straight across.

③ Remove calluses as soon as possible.

④ Apply lotion liberally, especially between the toes.

172. In assisting with planning Ms. Young's discharge, the nurse should insure that Ms. Young recognizes the common early symptoms of diabetic ketoacidosis, which include

① thirst and dry mucous membranes.

② cold, clammy skin and anxiety.

③ headache and weakness.

④ bulging of the eyeballs and dark amber urine.

Ms. Mary Varnick is a 25-year-old multigravida who is 8 months pregnant. She comes to the hospital and is admitted to the labor room with bright red vaginal bleeding. The physician suspects that Ms. Varnick may have placenta previa or abruptio placentae.

173. When Ms. Varnick is admitted, which of the following information should the nurse obtain **first**?

① Ms. Varnick's temperature and respiratory rate.

② Ms. Varnick's blood pressure and pulse rate.

③ Ms. Varnick's height and weight.

④ Ms. Varnick's laboratory results.

It is determined that Ms. Varnick has placenta previa, and a Cesarean section is performed under spinal anesthesia. A 4-lb (1,814-gm) girl is delivered and is transferred to the premature nursery, where she is placed in an incubator. Ms. Varnick is transferred from the recovery room to the postpartum unit.

174. In planning Ms. Varnick's postoperative care, which of the following measures should the nurse give **priority**?

① Instruct Ms. Varnick to lie flat in bed for at least eight hours.

② Allow Ms. Varnick to see her infant as soon as possible.

③ Record Ms. Varnick's intake and output.

④ Assess Ms. Varnick for muscle fatigue and ache.

175. An hour after Ms. Varnick is transferred to the postpartum unit, the nurse notes that her blood pressure reading has changed from 120/80 to 96/70 and that her abdominal dressings are dry. Which of the following actions should the nurse take **first**?

① Massage Ms. Varnick's uterine fundus.

② Elevate the foot of Ms. Varnick's bed.

③ Check Ms. Varnick's perineal pad.

④ Change Ms. Varnick's position.

176. On Ms. Varnick's fourth postpartum day, her lochia is bright red and moderate in amount. Which of the following actions should the nurse take?

① Encourage Ms. Varnick to increase her ambulation in order to aid involution.

② Have Ms. Varnick lie on her abdomen for about an hour in order to apply pressure to the uterus.

③ Record the observation.

④ Report the observation to the registered nurse in charge.

Mr. Jones, 75 years old, is seen in an outpatient clinic. He receives a diagnosis of herpes zoster involving the trigeminal nerve on the right side of his face. He has vesicles and a rash on his right cheek.

177. In collecting data from Mr. Jones, which of the following questions would be most important for the nurse to ask?

① "Have you been exposed to anyone with chickenpox?"

② "Do you have a history of developing canker sores?"

③ "Are you using a new shaving cream?"

④ "Have you ever had any allergic reactions to food?"

178. To relieve the discomfort Mr. Jones is experiencing, which of the following actions would be best for the nurse to include in the care plan?

① Debride the scabs.

② Clean the oozing discharge.

③ Apply petrolatum (Vaseline).

④ Apply cool compresses.

179. During the follow-up visit to the clinic, Mr. Jones asks, "Why do I still have pain where I had the herpes zoster?" Which of the following responses would be **most** appropriate for the nurse to make?

① "The pain is a manifestation of your fears."

② "The pain may persist for some time."

③ "The pain indicates an infection."

④ "The pain is evidence of muscle fatigue."

The following items are individual questions.

---

180. An adolescent client is seen in the out-patient clinic for a routine physical. Which of the following behaviors would the nurse expect to see?

① Conforming to adult standards.

② Worrying about athletic ability.

③ Having conflicts between dependence and independence.

④ Having definite vocational goals.

181. A client has been instructed to increase his intake of vitamin A. Which of the following foods should the nurse encourage him to eat?

① Roast beef and bacon.

② Corn and yellow beans.

③ Orange juice and bananas.

④ Carrots and sweet potatoes.

182. A client with newly diagnosed glaucoma says to the nurse, "I hope the treatment will improve my vision." Which of the following responses would be **best** for the nurse to make?

① "Blindness will eventually develop, but treatment will delay it."

② "Vision already lost cannot be restored, and continuous treatment is necessary to prevent further visual loss."

③ "Special eyeglasses will correct the visual impairment that occurs, but the lenses must be changed frequently."

④ "Surgery can restore lost vision and prevent recurrence of the disease."

183. A client is comatose. Which of the following measures is **essential** for the nurse to include in the care plan?

① Checking the client's blood pressure every two hours.

② Maintaining the client in a supported Fowler's position.

③ Turning the client from side to side at regular intervals.

④ Addressing the client in a loud tone.

184. A client has a liver biopsy. During the first few hours after the biopsy, the nurse should observe the client for which of the following complications?

① Gastric irritation.

② Infection.

③ Allergic reactions.

④ Hemorrhage.

185. An adult client has colostomy irrigations prescribed. Which of the following principles should the nurse include while reinforcing the teaching?

① Absorption of the irrigating fluid in the intestinal tract will be affected by the client's position.

② The pressure of the irrigating fluid in the intestinal tract will be determined by the height at which the fluid container is held.

③ The irrigating fluid dilates the blood vessels of the intestinal tract.

④ Manipulation of the irrigation catheter results in muscle spasm of the intestinal tract.

186. A client has severe preeclampsia. In monitoring the client, the nurse should be alert for which of the following symptoms?

① Ringing in the ears and rapid pulse.

② Elevated temperature and excitability.

③ Vomiting and excessive urination.

④ Persistent headache and blurred vision.

187. A newborn is diagnosed with hydrocephalus. Which of the following measures should the nurse include in the care plan?

① Measure abdominal girth daily.

② Change the baby's position every two hours.

③ Feed the baby on an established schedule.

④ Place the baby so the head is lower than the rest of the body.

188. A newborn has a cleft palate and is to be bottle fed. Which of the following measures would be **most** important for the nurse to take when feeding this infant?

① Applying elbow restraints to the infant prior to each feeding.

② Holding the infant in an upright position during feedings.

③ Giving the infant a small amount of sterile water after each feeding.

④ Feeding the infant small amounts frequently.

189.   An 11-year-old boy who is in a spica cast often eats too much and then complains of discomfort. Which of the following measures should the nurse take to prevent this problem?

① Give him smaller but more frequent meals.

② Continue to give him three meals a day, but give him smaller portions.

③ Restrict his fluid intake.

④ Encourage him to eat slowly and to alternate liquids with solids.

190.   A worker who is putting up a metal partition on the unit goes to a nurse on the floor and says that he just got a metal fragment in his eye. Which of the following actions by the nurse would demonstrate the **best** judgment?

① Suggest the man go see his personal physician.

② Irrigate the man's affected eye with sterile water.

③ Examine the man's affected eye.

④ Send the man to the emergency room.

191.   A client has had preoperative instructions on arm exercises prior to a modified radical mastectomy. While the nurse is reinforcing the teaching, the client says, ''Why will I have to exercise my arm after surgery when it will hurt?'' Which of the following responses would be **best** for the nurse to make?

① ''These exercises prevent stiffness of the shoulder and help you regain use of your arm.''

② ''Exercising the arm will actually decrease the amount of postoperative pain.''

③ ''This will eliminate the postoperative swelling that occurs at the incision.''

④ ''You are practicing now so that it won't be so uncomfortable for you later.''

192.   A client requires nasopharyngeal suctioning. Which of the following approaches would be **most** appropriate for the nurse to take when performing the procedure?

① Apply suction intermittently as the catheter is withdrawn.

② Apply suction continuously until the airway is clear.

③ Apply suction while administering oxygen.

④ Apply suction while irrigating with sterile normal saline.

193. The physician prescribes disulfiram (Antabuse) for a client. The nurse is reinforcing the teaching about the use of Antabuse. Which of the following statements, if made by the client, would indicate to the nurse that the teaching was successful?

① "The action of Antabuse continues for 72 hours after it is discontinued."

② "I should read labels carefully so I know what is in products that I eat."

③ "Antabuse should be taken at the same time everyday."

④ "The tablet should be crushed and mixed with liquid for optimal effectiveness."

194. When administering gastic gavage, the nurse should place the client in an upright position for the purpose of

① allowing the stomach to empty more easily.

② preventing aspiration and regurgitation.

③ allowing a normal position for eating.

④ preventing esophageal trauma.

195. Twelve hours after a client has abdominal surgery, the nurse listens for bowel sounds and determines that no bowel sounds are audible. Which of the following actions would be **most** appropriate for the nurse to take?

① Notify the nurse in charge regarding the absence of bowel sounds.

② Check for bowel sounds hourly.

③ Record the information on the client's chart.

④ Assist the client to ambulate.

196. A client is seen in the clinic two weeks after a skin graft. The client is concerned about the appearance and care of the donor site. After reviewing the care plan, which of the following responses by the nurse would be **most** appropriate?

① "Clean the area with soap and water every day and leave it alone."

② "Apply hydrogen peroxide to the area several times a day."

③ "Use an antibacterial soap and keep the area covered."

④ "Keep the area soft with lanolin cream or lotion."

197. The nurse is assisting a client who has diabetes mellitus to select his 1,800-calorie American Diabetes Association (ADA) diet. He states, "I don't like milk." Which of the following responses would be appropriate for the nurse to make?

① "You don't need to drink milk as long as your calories total the prescribed amount."

② "Your condition may become uncontrolled if you don't have a balanced diet that includes milk."

③ "Your insulin dosage will need to be adjusted if you don't include milk in your diet."

④ "You don't have to drink milk if you substitute another food of equal value."

198. The nurse observes a client with tuberculosis putting a soiled, disposable tissue in a pocket. Which of the following responses would be **most** appropriate for the nurse to make?

① "Let me get you a disposable bag for your used tissue."

② "Let me get you an emesis basin to dispose of your used tissue."

③ "Did you receive instructions about disposal of soiled tissues?"

④ "Can I help you dispose of your soiled tissue?"

199. A client with Alzheimer's disease repeatedly refuses to swallow an enteric-coated tablet. Which of the following approaches would be **most** appropriate for the nurse to take?

① Explain to the client the importance of taking the medication.

② Ask the nurse in charge for further instructions.

③ Crush the tablet and administer it with a small amount of food.

④ Withhold the tablet and attempt to administer it later.

200. A client with stiffness in the left hip is learning to use a walker. Which observation made by the nurse would indicate that the client understands the instructions given?

① The client advances the walker and steps forward alternating feet with each advancement.

② The client advances both feet, moves the walker forward, then moves both feet again.

③ The client advances the walker and steps forward with the left foot at the same time.

④ The client advances the right foot and then moves the walker forward, dragging the left foot.

201. A client is in deep sleep during the postictal state of a seizure. Which of the following measures should the nurse implement in caring for the client at this time?

① Perform neurological checks every 15 minutes.

② Position the client on either side.

③ Disturb the client as little as possible.

④ Notify the registered nurse in charge of the client's possible progression into a coma.

202. An adult client has sustained a concussion. When checking his level of consciousness, which of the following would indicate to the nurse that the client is stuporous?

① He is disoriented and has slow verbal response.

② He is difficult to arouse and has inappropriate verbal response.

③ He is unresponsive to painful stimuli.

④ He is responsive only to painful stimuli.

203. A postpartum client is taking a sitz bath. To **best** monitor the client's response during this treatment, the nurse should

① ask the client if she feels nauseated.

② check the client's pulse and skin color.

③ check the client's temperature and respirations.

④ ask the client if her symptoms are relieved.

204. A child is to have medication instilled in the ear. Which of the following is **essential** for the nurse to do in carrying out the procedure?

① Gain cooperation from the child's parents by explaining the procedure to them.

② Place the child in a side-lying position for 10 minutes after the instillation.

③ Straighten the ear canal by pulling the pinna downward and backward.

④ Cleanse the pinna with a small amount of distilled water prior to the instillation.

205. A client has organic brain syndrome. Which of the following approaches would be **most** appropriate for the nurse to include in the care plan?

① Carry out activities in the same order each day.

② Insist that the client focus conversation on present events.

③ Provide a variety of activities for the client.

④ Introduce the client to all nursing staff.

206. A client has 0.08 mg of digoxin (Lanoxin) ordered. The bottle contains 0.05 mg of the drug in 1 cc of solution. How much solution should the nurse prepare for administration?

① 0.06 cc

② 0.6 cc

③ 1.6 cc

④ 2.6 cc

207. A client has a history of seizures. Which of the following should the nurse have available?

① Oxygen and suction equipment.

② Leather restraints.

③ Cardiac monitor.

④ Venous cutdown set and oxygen.

208. Discharge teaching has been completed with the parents of a 3-year-old male hemophiliac. Which comments made by the parents would indicate to the nurse an understanding of the long-term implications of the child's health problem?

① "Doing active range of motion activities with him will help prevent contractures."

② "We will provide a warm indulgent environment to promote his emotional development."

③ "Overprotection can interfere with his emotional and physical development."

④ "He will limit his own physical activity which is typical of children with his condition."

209. A mother asks the nurse why her 2-year-old daughter has developed otitis media. Which of the following responses by the nurse would be **best**?

① "The eustachian tube is short and wide in children, predisposing them to infections."

② "The causative organism is part of the normal flora in the throat of children."

③ "The external ear is less effective in children in resisting the entrance of organisms."

④ "The inner ear in children is markedly immature, so they get more infections than adults."

210. In evaluating the effects of a prescribed expectorant, the nurse should expect the client to exhibit which of the following effects?

① Cough suppression.

② Bronchial relaxation.

③ Reduced viscosity of respiratory secretions.

④ Decreased production of respiratory secretions.

211. In assessing a 68-year-old client, which of the following comments made by the client would indicate to the nurse normal changes associated with the aging process?

① "I seldom need to use a cover at night."

② "I think I'm shorter than I used to be."

③ "I can still see as well with these glasses as I could 10 years ago."

④ "It takes me a while to find a comfortable position to sleep in."

212. A client with osteoarthritis questions the need for physical therapy. Which of the following responses by the nurse would be **most** appropriate?

① "Physical therapy will gradually increase the stress tolerance of your joints."

② "Physical therapy will prevent further destruction of joint tissues."

③ "Physical therapy will promote tightening of joint tendons."

④ "Physical therapy will maintain as near normal joint function as possible."

213. In planning care for a client with a diagnosis of infectious hepatitis (Type A), which of the following nursing measures is **essential**?

① Serving food on disposable dishes.

② Wearing a face mask while providing care.

③ Carrying out procedures for enteric precautions.

④ Modifying procedures for discarding used syringes and needles.

214. In reinforcing teaching with a client diagnosed with hepatitis (Type A), the nurse determines that the teaching has been successful if the client refrains from

① smoking.

② eating fried foods.

③ donating blood.

④ exercising strenuously.

215. A client with thrombophlebitis is placed on bed rest. The client asks why bed rest is necessary. Which of the following responses by the nurse would be **best**?

① "Bed rest promotes venous pressure in the extremities."

② "Bed rest improves the venous circulation."

③ "Bed rest minimizes the potential for release of a blood clot."

④ "Bed rest prevents blood clot formation in the unaffected extremity."

216. In evaluating the effectiveness of heparin sodium, U.S.P. therapy, the nurse would monitor the results of which of the following laboratory tests?

① Prothrombin time.

② Partial thromboplastin time.

③ Red cell fragility.

④ Platelet count.

217. A client is unable to produce enough sputum for a specimen. Which of the following measures would be **best** for the nurse to implement to help the client expectorate the sputum?

① Apply external heat to the chest for a few minutes.

② Have the client drink a large glass of cool water.

③ Place the client in high Fowler's position.

④ Have the client breathe humidified air.

218. The nursing diagnosis, activity intolerance related to decreased oxygenation, is established for a client. To promote activity tolerance in the client, the nurse should plan to

① have the client decide which activities will be done for the day.

② complete all care at one time to avoid disturbing the client later.

③ space nursing activities to allow the client frequent rest periods.

④ suggest ways in which the client can participate in performing care.

219. To reinforce teaching regarding prevention of infections in a client with a urinary catheter, the nurse should emphasize which of the following?

① Encourage the client to eat a balanced diet.

② Advise the client to drink liberal amounts of fluid.

③ Tell the client to drink at least one glass of cranberry juice per day.

④ Direct the client to keep the drainage bag at bladder level.

220. A client is admitted to the hospital with a diagnosis of renal calculus. Before admission orders are received, which of the following actions would be **most** important for the nurse to initiate?

① Provide a quiet environment for the client.

② Strain all the client's urine.

③ Advise the client to remain on bed rest.

④ Restrict the client's food and fluids.

221. Which of the following signs, if observed by the nurse in a postpartal woman, would indicate the presence of an abnormality?

① A chill shortly after delivery.

② A pulse rate of 60 the morning after delivery.

③ Urinary output of 3,000 ml the second day after delivery.

④ Oral temperature of 101°F (38.3°C) the third day after delivery.

222. A client has hypertension. Which of the following findings by the nurse would constitute a significant index of hypertension?

① Pulse deficit of 10 beats per minute.

② Regular pulse of 90 beats per minute.

③ Systolic pressure fluctuating between 150 and 160 mm Hg.

④ Diastolic pressure sustained at greater than 90 mm Hg.

223. A 2-month-old infant is brought to the well-baby clinic and is given a diphtheria, tetanus, pertussis (DTP) injection and trivalent oral polio vaccine (TOPV). Which of the following would be **most** important for the nurse to reinforce with the infant's parent during the visit?

① The infant may become fussy and irritable.

② The infant needs to return in two months for repeat immunization.

③ The parent should keep a record of all of the infant's immunizations.

④ The parent should seek treatment if the infant sleeps excessively.

224. A client has a positive skin test for tuberculosis. This would **most** likely indicate to the nurse that

① the client is free of tuberculosis infection.

② the client has an active case of tuberculosis.

③ the client is immune to tuberculosis and cannot contract the disease.

④ the client has been previously exposed to the tubercle bacillus.

225. A loud argument between two elderly roommates in a long-term care facility leaves hostile feelings between them. One of the roommates threatens to leave the facility if something is not done about the situation. Which of the following measures would be **most** appropriate for the nurse to take?

① Talk with the clients to gain insight into their conflict.

② Move one of the roommates to a different room.

③ Create different diversional activities for each roommate.

④ Have a psychiatric nurse meet with the clients.

226. The nurse begins resuscitative measures on a 4-year-old who has stopped breathing. To administer effective breaths for the child, the nurse should

① pinch off the nares and hyperextend his neck.

② pinch off the nares and slightly tilt his head.

③ lift his jaw and breathe into his nares.

④ encircle and breathe into his mouth and nares.

227. Nitroglycerin ointment 2% (Nitro-Bid) is prescribed for a client. When administering the medication, the nurse should

① apply the ointment with the fingertips.

② rub the ointment into the area thoroughly.

③ place the dose-determining applicator over the medication.

④ cover the site with plastic wrap.

228. A client's wife comes to the hospice every day to visit her husband. To provide support to the client's wife, it would be **most** appropriate for the nurse to

① suggest to the client's wife that she attend a group for families of dying clients.

② ask the client's wife how she would like to help in her husband's care.

③ suggest to the client's wife that she visit the social worker.

④ have the client bathed and groomed in time for his wife's arrival each morning.

229. A child is admitted with injuries that are suspected of being inflicted by her parents. A nursing assistant on the unit says to the nurse, ''Every time I see that child's parents, I see red. How could any adult, least of all parents, deliberately hurt a child?'' Which of the following responses by the nurse would be **most** helpful to the nursing assistant?

① ''Making judgments about parent's actions is not appropriate for nursing personnel.''

② ''You must not let the parents know how you feel.''

③ ''It is an upsetting situation, isn't it?''

④ ''There is no legal proof of abuse at this time.''

230. A client with terminal cancer is admitted to a long-term care facility. The client's prescriptions include morphine sulfate (Roxanol) 30 mg by mouth every two hours. Which of the following understandings regarding this prescription would be correct?

① The dose is too large.

② The prescribed period of frequency is too short.

③ The dose is too small.

④ The prescription is appropriate.

231. On the second day following a client's colectomy, the physician prescribes a dressing change. The client's incision is large and has two Penrose drains. Which of the following information would be **essential** for the nurse to include when recording the procedure?

① Amount of drainage, degree of wound healing, and client's tolerance of procedure.

② Condition of wound and surrounding tissue, length of procedure, and type of dressing used.

③ Time dressing is changed, description of wound, and the amount of drainage.

④ Presence of drainage, type of dressing used, and client's response.

232. A mother calls a neighbor who is a nurse and says that her toddler ate an unknown plant in the backyard and now appears ill. In addition to telling the mother to call the poison control center immediately, which of the following would be appropriate for the nurse to say?

① "Obtain a urine specimen from the child."

② "Have the child drink an ounce of mineral oil."

③ "Put the child to bed and elevate his extremities."

④ "Make the child vomit and save the vomitus."

233. A client is to receive a rectal suppository. Which of the following is the **best** position for the nurse to ask the client to assume?

① Turn to the right side with the upper leg flexed.

② Turn to the left side with the right knee flexed.

③ Assume a comfortable position on either side.

④ Assume a prone position with either leg flexed.

234. The wife of a client with congestive heart failure (CHF) expresses concern over the danger of her husband's condition. She tells the nurse, "I am so afraid he will stop breathing when we are alone at home. I know CPR, but I wish I had someone to assist me with it." Which of the following responses would be **best** for the nurse to make?

① "Lay rescuers are now advised to administer one-person CPR even when two rescuers are present."

② "Sixty to seventy percent of sudden deaths caused by cardiac arrest occur at home."

③ "Neighbors are often willing to learn how to provide assistance with cardiac arrest."

④ "One-person CPR attempts, though acceptable, are not as effective as two-person CPR attempts."

235. A client who has genital herpes has been instructed in methods to prevent transmission. Upon entering the client's room, the nurse observes the client's friend coming out of the bathroom. Which of the following actions would be **essential** for the nurse to take first?

① Report the incident to the nurse in charge.

② Record the incident in the nurses' notes.

③ Reinforce precaution instructions to the client and the client's friend.

④ Discuss precaution instructions with the client after the friend leaves.

236. After receiving diet and fitness instruction, an obese client asks the nurse to select an appropriate exercise program. Which of the following questions should the nurse ask to **best** assist the client in a selection?

① "Can you join a local fitness center?"

② "What type of exercise do you enjoy?"

③ "Will your friends be exercising with you?"

④ "How important is rapid weight loss to you?"

237. A client in a long-term care facility has an artificial eye that will be inserted after the eye socket is free from infection. Which of the following would be the **best** site for storing this item until it can be inserted?

① In a labeled container of water in the nightstand.

② In a labeled container in the nurses' station.

③ In a labeled container in the medicine room.

④ In a labeled container of sterile saline in the nightstand.

238. The nurse is reinforcing the instructions given to a hospitalized client scheduled for external radiation therapy. Which of the following statements made by the client would indicate to the nurse that the teaching has been successful?

① "I will be placed in isolation for the duration of my therapy."

② "I will be taken to another area of the hospital to receive my treatments."

③ "My visitors will be restricted until my therapy is complete."

④ "My room will be radioactive from the treatment."

239. A client has undergone a cardiac catheterization using the left femoral artery. For the first few hours after the procedure, which of the following measures would be **essential** for the nurse to implement?

① Keep the head of the client's bed elevated 30 degrees.

② Encourage the client to cough forcefully at regular intervals.

③ Check the client's temperature every hour.

④ Take the client's pulse frequently in the extremity used for the insertion.

240. When irrigating a draining wound with a sterile saline solution, which of the following sequences would be **most** appropriate for the nurse to use?

① Wash hands, prepare sterile field, and remove soiled dressing.

② Prepare sterile field, put on sterile gloves, and remove soiled dressing.

③ Pour solution, wash hands, and remove soiled dressing.

④ Remove soiled dressing, flush wound, and wash hands.

Answers

PART I

PART II

Answers, Part I

Item #	Correct Answer	Rationale
1.	④	Angina pectoris occurs when the blood supply to the heart is inadequate to meet the demand of the heart muscle. Stress will constrict the blood vessels, reducing the blood supply. Pain results when lack of oxygenation of the heart muscle exists. *Nursing Process:* Collecting data *Client Need:* Physiological integrity
2.	②	Nitroglycerin improves coronary blood flow by dilating coronary arteries and intercoronary collateral vessels. It relieves the pain of angina in one to two minutes. *Nursing Process:* Evaluating *Client Need:* Physiological integrity
3.	③	Fear of pain is a normal reaction for Mr. Samm. The pain of myocardial infarction is so severe the client often believes that he is dying. *Nursing Process:* Evaluating *Client Need:* Physiological integrity
4.	④	Oxygen supports combustion. Therefore, necessary precautions such as no smoking signs should be posted in the room and outside the room. *Nursing Process:* Implementing *Client Need:* Safe, effective care environment
5.	④	Hemorrhage is the principal adverse reaction of anticoagulant therapy. Therefore, the client should be checked for hematuria by hemostix. *Nursing Process:* Collecting data *Client Need:* Physiological integrity
6.	③	Fresh fruits and vegetables have less sodium than processed foods. *Nursing Process:* Implementing *Client Need:* Physiological integrity
7.	③	Promoting rest and relaxation is a major therapy goal since relaxation decreases oxygen demands. When the nurse suggests any diversion, the need for relaxation should be considered. *Nursing Process:* Planning *Client Need:* Safe, effective care environment
8.	①	Recommending a priest to Ms. Samm is the most appropriate response. A priest can address Ms. Samm's worries about frightening her husband. *Nursing Process:* Implementing *Client Need:* Health promotion/maintenance
9.	③	The most accurate description of a thready pulse is rapid and weak. Another description of a thready pulse is fine and scarcely perceptible. *Nursing Process:* Evaluating *Client Need:* Physiological integrity

Item #	Correct Answer	Rationale
10.	④	Cheyne-Stokes respirations are defined as alternating periods of apnea and hyperpnea. Apnea lasting 10 to 60 seconds is followed by gradually increasing and decreasing respirations. *Nursing Process:* Collecting data *Client Need:* Physiological integrity
11.	④	The appearance of Mr. Samm's body will be important to his family. Therefore, the body should be arranged to look as natural as possible, as if the deceased person is sleeping. *Nursing Process:* Implementing *Client Need:* Physiological integrity
12.	②	Bleeding may continue and cause severe hemorrhage until all products of conception have been expelled. The number of pads used and the amount and type of drainage should be recorded. *Nursing Process:* Planning *Client Need:* Physiological integrity
13.	①	Seconal is a short-acting barbiturate which works as a central nervous system depressant. It is administered to Ms. Miller in preparation for surgery to produce mild sedation, thus reducing her level of anxiety. *Nursing Process:* Evaluating *Client Need:* Physiological integrity
14.	②	An operative consent is a legal document that protects the client and the hospital. The registered nurse in charge must be told of its absence since she is responsible for management of client care and insuring that consent is obtained before surgery. *Nursing Process:* Implementing *Client Need:* Safe, effective care environment
15.	④	Atropine sulfate reduces salivation and bronchial secretions. It is administered preoperatively to lessen secretions in the upper respiratory tract and thus decrease the possibility of aspiration during surgery. *Nursing Process:* Evaluating *Client Need:* Physiological integrity
16.	①	4,500,000 to 5,000,000 cu. mm. is in the normal range for red blood cells in a healthy adult female. Since 2,500,000 is significantly lower than normal, this must be brought to the attention of the registered nurse in charge so further instructions for care may be obtained. *Nursing Process:* Implementing *Client Need:* Physiological integrity
17.	③	Iron preparations may be irritating to the stomach lining and cause nausea. It is best to take iron immediately after meals since food in the stomach prevents the preparation from coming into direct contact with the gastric mucosa and causing irritation. *Nursing Process:* Implementing *Client Need:* Physiological integrity

Item #	Correct Answer	Rationale
18.	①	All forms of leukemia are characterized by weakness, fatigue, anorexia, weight loss, anemia, enlarged body organs, and hemorrhage. *Nursing Process:* Collecting data *Client Need:* Physiological integrity
19.	④	A client may have an allergic reaction to receiving a blood transfusion. The blood may contain antibodies that trigger this reaction. Administration of an antihistamine, such as diphenhydramine hydrochloride, is a method to minimize such an allergic reaction. *Nursing Process:* Evaluating *Client Need:* Physiological integrity
20.	②	Gums bleed frequently in patients with leukemia due to lowered platelet counts. Mouth care must be done, but only with soft bristled toothbrushes. The taste of blood can be relieved by rinsing with normal saline or diluted solution of hydrogen peroxide. Mouthwash contains alcohol which may be drying and irritating. *Nursing Process:* Planning *Client Need:* Physiological integrity
21.	③	An antiemetic given to Mr. Gayle one half hour before a scheduled meal will take effect by the time the meal is served. Relief of nausea will make Mr. Gayle more interested in eating. Small, bland feedings are least likely to provoke indigestion or nausea. *Nursing Process:* Planning *Client Need:* Physiological integrity
22.	②	The nurse's acceptance of Mr. Gayle's mood identifies it as a valid response to his illness and prognosis. This will help with the client's own acceptance of his response as normal. *Nursing Process:* Planning *Client Need:* Health promotion/maintenance
23.	①	Mr. Gayle's comments to the nurse are statements of his understanding of his illness. The nurse's response should confirm his realistic statements without giving false hope or trying to distract him. *Nursing Process:* Implementing *Client Need:* Health promotion/maintenance
24.	③	Mr. Gayle has leukemia and has already had an episode of bleeding from his gums. It is important to maintain his circulatory status and blood clotting mechanisms. Aspirin interferes with prothrombin formation and ingestion of aspirin may lead to another bleeding episode. *Nursing Process:* Implementing *Client Need:* Health promotion/maintenance
25.	②	The nurse should acknowledge June's anxiety and allow June to explore the options her physician has already identified. *Nursing Process:* Implementing *Client Need:* Psychosocial integrity

Item #	Correct Answer	Rationale
26.	②	The nurse mentions something that has been observed about the client. The technique lets clients know that the listener is observing facts about them and is hearing what they are trying to express. *Nursing Process:* Implementing *Client Need:* Psychosocial integrity
27.	④	In the immediate postoperative period, bleeding is the principal concern. Although position and control of infection are important, they are not a priority at this time. *Nursing Process:* Implementing *Client Need:* Physiological integrity
28.	④	A grief reaction should be expected following an amputation. "Can you tell me what's bothering you, June?" acknowledges June's grief and is not judgmental or punitive. *Nursing Process:* Implementing *Client Need:* Psychosocial integrity
29.	①	Vitamin C and protein are needed to promote adequate wound healing and should therefore be plentiful in June's diet. *Nursing Process:* Planning *Client Need:* Physiological integrity
30.	③	Adolescents need the social approval of their peer group, and June's concern about her friends' acceptance will cause added difficulty in her adjustment to the amputation. *Nursing Process:* Planning *Client Need:* Health promotion/maintenance
31.	②	The nurse should be sensitive to the underlying reason for June's outburst. June is scared, unhappy, and depressed. All other answers are wrong because they do not acknowledge June's feelings and instead require June to understand the pressures of the nurse's job. *Nursing Process:* Implementing *Client Need:* Psychosocial integrity
32.	③	Phantom-limb is both physiological and psychological in origin. Pain medication is the priority. Encouraging June to express her feelings is a useful adjunct to medication. Exercise and elevation will not help. *Nursing Process:* Implementing *Client Need:* Physiological integrity
33.	③	It is common for elderly clients who have lost a spouse to miss the physical contact and emotional support the spouse formerly provided. Mr. Cone and Ms. Foster are responding to one another's genuine sexual and emotional needs. It is important for the nursing staff to respect these needs before arriving at a plan of action. *Nursing Process:* Planning *Client Need:* Health promotion/maintenance

Item #	Correct Answer	Rationale
34.	③	Mr. Cone's repeated discussions of his child rearing methods illustrate his uncertainty about them. He continues to be uncertain whether he always made appropriate decisions, and wonders whether his children suffered from them. *Nursing Process:* Evaluating *Client Need:* Health promotion/maintenance
35.	②	Coronary artery disease is considered to be related to a person's daily life and habits. Weight is also thought to have an effect on the development of coronary artery disease. An overweight person subjected to stress can be a candidate for developing coronary artery disease. A diet high in saturated fats is also a risk factor. *Nursing Process:* Implementing *Client Need:* Health promotion/maintenance
36.	②	An EKG has no preparation, no physical exercise requirements, and no adverse side effects. *Nursing Process:* Implementing *Client Need:* Safe, effective care environment
37.	②	Because Mr. Cone and Ms. Foster are involved in a relationship, it is natural for Ms. Foster to be concerned about Mr. Cone. Arranging for Ms. Foster to visit will reassure her that Mr. Cone is stable. *Nursing Process:* Implementing *Client Need:* Health promotion/maintenance
38.	③	Symptoms of digitalis toxicity include: decreased pulse rate, cardiac arrhythmias, nausea, vomiting, loss of appetite, abdominal cramps, and visual disturbance. Of the choices here, nausea is the only one recognized as a symptom of digitalis toxicity. *Nursing Process:* Evaluating *Client Need:* Health promotion/maintenance
39.	①	After bronchoscopy the nurse must determine the return of the "gag" reflex before the client is allowed to take fluid. If the gag reflex is not present, Ms. Jacobson could aspirate when she takes a drink. *Nursing Process:* Implementing *Client Need:* Safe, effective care environment
40.	②	A serious complication of bronchoscopy would be swelling due to the trauma of the procedure. The first symptom the client would experience would be difficulty in breathing. *Nursing Process:* Collecting data *Client Need:* Physiological integrity
41.	④	Before any action can be taken, the nurse must determine what Ms. Jacobson is feeling. Listening attentively will provide emotional support, as well as allowing the nurse to discover whether Ms. Jacobson needs additional help or information. *Nursing Process:* Implementing *Client Need:* Safe, effective care environment

Item #	Correct Answer	Rationale
42.	①	A chest tube is inserted into the pleural space to allow for the drainage of fluid and air and to maintain a negative pressure. *Nursing Process:* Implementing *Client Need:* Safe, effective care environment
43.	③	Fluctuation is expected to occur with each respiration. If fluctuation does not occur it indicates that something is plugging the tubing or the lung has reinflated. *Nursing Process:* Collecting data *Client Need:* Physiological integrity
44.	③	Tomato juice contains high amounts of vitamin C. Vitamin C promotes wound healing. *Nursing Process:* Implementing *Client Need:* Physiological integrity
45.	④	A complaint of pain can have many causes. The nurse should not assume that the client's pain originates from the incision. The exact nature and location of pain should be assessed. First the nurse must determine the specifics by asking Ms. Jacobson to describe her pain in more detail. *Nursing Process:* Collecting data *Client Need:* Physiological integrity
46.	②	Offering Ms. Jacobson fluids every hour will provide her with a graphic reminder of the importance of adequate fluid intake. In addition, small amounts will not overwhelm Ms. Jacobson, and she is more likely to be able to take the prescribed amount of fluid. *Nursing Process:* Implementing *Client Need:* Physiological integrity
47.	③	Interviewing the client is one method of collecting data for the development of the nursing care plan. The client is usually the best source for information about his patterns of coping with activities of daily living. *Nursing Process:* Collecting data *Client Need:* Safe, effective care environment
48.	②	The first symptoms of Parkinson's disease are usually tremors which tend to become aggravated by stress and anxiety. The client's care should include ways to reduce anxiety-producing situations. By allowing enough time to perform activities, the client will not be rushed, and stress will be lessened. *Nursing Process:* Planning *Client Need:* Health promotion/maintenance
49.	①	Drug therapy is used for symptomatic treatment, because there is no cure for this disease. Levodopa has been used successfully in reducing tremors and rigidity. *Nursing Process:* Evaluating *Client Need:* Physiological integrity

Item #	Correct Answer	Rationale
50.	④	One of the goals in caring for a client with Parkinson's disease is to prolong independence. Therefore, Mr. Walker is encouraged to carry out his usual activities of daily living. *Nursing Process:* Implementing *Client Need:* Health promotion/maintenance
51.	④	It is natural for Mr. Walker to be frustrated by his inability to work. The nurse might suggest that he rest briefly and then return to his manuscript, thus expressing confidence that he is still capable of independence and productive work. *Nursing Process:* Evaluating *Client Need:* Psychosocial integrity
52.	①	As the prostate gland enlarges it puts pressure on the urethra causing urinary stasis, recurring infections, frequent urination, nocturia, and dysuria. *Nursing Process:* Collecting data *Client Need:* Safe, effective care environment
53.	①	An appropriate response would be for the nurse to check to see whether Mr. Little's minister is coming. If not, another visit can be arranged. Answers 2 and 3 are empty promises and a way of putting Mr. Little off. *Nursing Process:* Implementing *Client Need:* Psychosocial integrity
54.	③	Continuous bladder irrigations require a steady flow of fluids into the bladder. Fluid entering the bladder and fluid draining from the bladder should be in appropriate proportions. Patency must be checked frequently to prevent distention of the client's bladder. *Nursing Process:* Implementing *Client Need:* Physiological integrity
55.	③	A clogged urinary catheter would be an obvious cause of increased pain after a transurethral prostatectomy. Such a clog could be due to the presence of a blood clot. The correct response is to check Mr. Little's urinary drainage apparatus. *Nursing Process:* Implementing *Client Need:* Physiological integrity
56.	①	Without continuous irrigations, the urine will be bright red. With continuous irrigations, the urine is usually slightly pink or clear. *Nursing Process:* Collecting data *Client Need:* Physiological integrity
57.	③	After a period of bed rest Mr. Little will need time to adjust to an upright position. Sitting on the edge of the bed will aid in this adjustment. It would be inappropriate to clamp the urethral catheter. *Nursing Process:* Implementing *Client Need:* Physiological integrity

Item #	Correct Answer	Rationale
58.	①	The presence of a urinary catheter dilates the urinary sphincter. After the catheter is removed, it would not be unusual for dribbling of urine to occur. The other options would indicate a problem. *Nursing Process:* Evaluating *Client Need:* Health promotion/maintenance
59.	④	The primary instructions given after a transurethral prostatectomy are: void whenever there is an urge, avoid straining during defecation, avoid constipation, avoid sitting, eat adequate fiber, and take adequate fluids. *Nursing Process:* Implementing *Client Need:* Health promotion/maintenance
60.	③	Although a heat source is usually wrapped in a towel, it is essential that the temperature of the heat source be checked prior to application. If the source is too hot a towel will not prevent a burn. *Nursing Process:* Implementing *Client Need:* Physiological integrity
61.	②	Demerol is a central nervous system depressant. Respiratory distress could occur after administration. Therefore Ms. Kerr's respiratory rate must be checked beforehand so that a baseline can be determined. If the rate is too low the drug should be withheld. *Nursing Process:* Collecting data *Client Need:* Physiological integrity
62.	③	Flexion of the spine should be avoided. The correct way for the nurse to arrange the bedpan is to turn Ms. Kerr to her side, put the bedpan in place, and return her to back-lying position on the bedpan. Use of overbed trapeze is contraindicated.
63.	③	Accurate assessment of changes in skin color cannot be made if a client has makeup on. Established preoperative routines require removal of makeup in order to provide safe care. *Nursing Process:* Implementing *Client Need:* Safe, effective care environment
64.	①	The development of shock is characterized by a dropping blood pressure and a rising pulse. Therefore a blood pressure of 100/60 and a pulse of 120 would signal shock in Ms. Kerr. *Nursing Process:* Evaluating *Client Need:* Physiological integrity
65.	①	Both during and after a period of immobility, the client is at risk for development of thrombophlebitis. The correct nursing intervention is to instruct Ms. Kerr to remain in bed and report the symptom to the registered nurse in charge. Ambulation and massage could loosen the possible clot, causing an embolus. *Nursing Process:* Implementing *Client Need:* Physiological integrity

Item #	Correct Answer	Rationale
66.	④	During the night it is dark; there is a lack of stimulation and a lack of personnel to establish a relationship between time and place. Mr. Anderman will be most confused when awakening in the middle of the night. *Nursing Process:* Planning *Client Need:* Psychosocial integrity
67.	②	To insure that Mr. Anderman's nutritional requirements are met, his ability to chew food must be assessed. *Nursing Process:* Collecting data *Client Need:* Physiological integrity
68.	④	Overall nutritional needs of the elderly are essentially the same as other adults, except that their caloric needs diminish because they are simply maintaining a stable body structure. *Nursing Process:* Planning *Client Need:* Physiological integrity
69.	②	Placing a light blanket over Mr. Anderman's feet is the simplest and safest method of keeping them warm. *Nursing Process:* Implementing *Client Need:* Physiological integrity
70.	②	Clamping the tubing and instructing Ms. Evan to take deep breaths is the first appropriate intervention. This may help her hold the solution because it relaxes the abdominal muscles. *Nursing Process:* Implementing *Client Need:* Physiological integrity
71.	③	The purpose of the preoperative medication is to relax the client, alleviate anxiety, and permit smooth induction of anesthesia prior to surgery. Therefore, Ms. Evan should not be disturbed after the preoperative medication. Her morning care should be completed before the medication is given. *Nursing Process:* Planning *Client Need:* Safe, effective care environment
72.	④	Inspecting Ms. Evan's dressing for bleeding should be the nurse's next action. External bleeding, which could occur within the first 24 hours after surgery, would be detected by checking the dressing. The other actions should be done, but vital signs and checking for bleeding are most important. *Nursing Process:* Implementing *Client Need:* Physiological integrity
73.	③	Mouth care will prevent dryness and discomfort for Ms. Evan by keeping the mucous membrane of the mouth moist. *Nursing Process:* Planning *Client Need:* Physiological integrity

Item #	Correct Answer	Rationale
74.	④	Venous stasis could lead to serious postoperative complications such as the formation of venous thrombosis. Exercising the legs helps to prevent this complication. *Nursing Process:* Planning *Client Need:* Physiological integrity
75.	②	The nurse should keep communication open, despite the fact Ms. Turner is being difficult. By responding with, ''You think I'm talking down to you,'' the nurse shows respect for Ms. Turner's feelings and allows her to calm down. The other responses are unnecessarily argumentative. *Nursing Process:* Implementing *Client Need:* Safe, effective care environment
76.	①	In order to remove gas and fluids from the stomach, the physician will usually prescribe gastric decompression by use of a nasogastric tube. This procedure prevents nausea, vomiting, and distention that could occur after surgery due to decreased peristalsis. *Nursing Process:* Implementing *Client Need:* Physiological integrity
77.	①	It would be most important to have Ms. Turner breathe deeply and cough in order to prevent postoperative complications such as atelectasis and pneumonia. Improving respiratory function is the most important goal of postoperative care. *Nursing Process:* Planning *Client Need:* Physiological integrity
78.	①	Most ileostomy clients worry about odor control and bowel excretion. They will take the attitude of the nurse as an example of the way other people will react. By not showing distaste when changing Ms. Turner's ileostomy bag, the nurse is teaching Ms. Turner not to be embarrassed about caring for her ileostomy. *Nursing Process:* Implementing *Client Need:* Health promotion/maintenance
79.	③	The ostomy visitor will usually check with the nurse about any specifics to be discussed. Then the visitor should be introduced to the client. After the introduction, the client and the visitor should be allowed a quiet, private visit. *Nursing Process:* Implementing *Client Need:* Health promotion/maintenance
80.	④	The simplest explanation for Ms. Turner's lack of appetite is that the meals don't appeal to her. The nurse should ask if she likes her food before assuming the problem is bigger than it really is. Explaining the need for proper nutrition should be part of the nursing care plan but is not the most appropriate action at this time. *Nursing Process:* Implementing *Client Need:* Physiological integrity

Item #	Correct Answer	Rationale

81. ③ In an emergency situation, the first action taken must be the determination and maintenance of a patent airway. Without adequate respiratory function, all other measures are futile.
Nursing Process: Implementing
Client Need: Physiological integrity

82. ① The client is in the lateral decubitus position with knees drawn up and chin down to increase the space between the vertebrae.
Nursing Process: Implementing
Client Need: Safe, effective care environment

83. ② To insure a safe spinal tap, the client must remain perfectly still. The primary function of the nurse is to help the patient remain motionless throughout the procedure. The nurse should explain the procedure to the client before it begins. Labels should be prepared prior to the procedure.
Nursing Process: Implementing
Client Need: Safe, effective care environment

84. ④ Accurate observation, description, and documentation of the seizure and their progression are necessary to classify the type of seizure. Restriction of movement may result in broken bones.
Nursing Process: Implementing
Client Need: Physiological integrity

85. ③ Clinical signs of increased intracranial pressure may include: headache, vomiting, changes in level of consciousness, motor function, respirations, pupils, ocular movements, and vital signs.
Nursing Process: Collecting data
Client Need: Physiological integrity

86. ③ Alzheimer's clients should have limits set on their behavior. Firmly but kindly identifying what behavior is unacceptable causes less agitation than restraint or reprimand. Leaving the patient causes them to feel rejection and they may never "calm" down.
Nursing Process: Implementing
Client Need: Psychosocial integrity

87. ④ Current thought on Alzheimer's indicates that overstimulation increases agitation in clients with the disorder. Yet stimulation is necessary to provide some reality orientation. Restraining only increases agitation. The room should be brightly lit in the day time and there should be sufficient light at night to help the client identify the surroundings.
Nursing Process: Planning
Client Need: Psychosocial integrity

Item #	Correct Answer	Rationale

88. ② Exercise is the only preventive measure for contractions. Exercise keeps tendons, ligaments, and muscle flexible. In a client with existing contractions, the exercising is done to the limit of their contractions. Range of motion may be easier to accomplish after relaxation of the joint in a warm bath but daily bathing is contraindicated for fragile, geriatric skin.
Nursing Process: Implementing
Client Need: Physiological integrity

89. ① Nothing should be placed in the mouth of a confused client, yet the most accurate temperature possible is needed. Thus, the temperature should be taken rectally. The apical pulse is the most accurate.
Nursing Process: Implementing
Client Need: Physiological integrity

90. ① Doing postural drainage prior to meals causes the patient to cough up sputum during mealtime which is unpleasant. Doing postural drainage immediately after meals causes pressure on a full stomach. The most beneficial times are in the morning to clear secretions collected during the night and at night to make the patient comfortable for sleep.
Nursing Process: Implementing
Client Need: Physiological integrity

91. ③ The greatest degree of vulnerability for the client with a walker is to the back where the walker is open. The nurse must be able to see ahead of the patient, thus the greatest degree of safety is provided when the nurse walks behind but slightly to the side of a client ambulating with a walker.
Nursing Process: Implementing
Client Need: Physiological integrity

92. ④ Adaptation depends on the ability to overcome obstacles and choose those activities within the person's capabilities. Distractors 2 and 3 show a reluctance to participate in activities of daily living. The best adaptation is shown when the person acknowledges the deficit and chooses an appropriate lower level physical activity which still challenges mental activity.
Nursing Process: Evaluating
Client Need: Health promotion/maintenance

93. ④ The whirlpool tub assists in promoting circulation, as well as giving the resident a general feeling of cleanliness and well-being. Her anxiety results from fear of being left alone and "something happening" to her. While encouraging her to do as much as possible for herself, the nurse should remain in sight to assist when needed.
Nursing Process: Implementing
Client Need: Physiological integrity

Item #	Correct Answer	Rationale
94.	②	Stress incontinence can be relieved to some degree by teaching the client how to strengthen the pubococcygeal muscle. Although bathing and protection of clothing are important, they do not address rehabilitation for the problem. *Nursing Process:* Implementing *Client Need:* Health promotion/maintenance
95.	③	With aging, deep levels of sleep are less prominent and brief arousals more frequent. Total sleep time is not reduced from young adulthood. *Nursing Process:* Evaluating *Client Need:* Health promotion/maintenance
96.	③	The client must contact the physician immediately if nausea or vomiting is experienced because this raises intraocular pressure. Discomfort (not pain) is normal. The client may sleep on his or her back or unoperated side. Straining during bowel movements is contraindicated. *Nursing Process:* Evaluating *Client Need:* Health promotion/maintenance
97.	①	Arterial blood supply is very superficial at groin and axillae. Cool, moist packs would be most effective at these points. *Nursing Process:* Implementing *Client Need:* Physiological integrity
98.	③	The bladder lies in the anterior of the pelvis and, if full, could interfere with assessment of other pelvic organs. An empty bladder also allows for a more relaxed client. *Nursing Process:* Implementing *Client Need:* Safe, effective care environment
99.	③	Delirium tremens are characterized by progressive disorientation to time and place. The client will be restless and confused. As the condition advances, the client becomes agitated and combative and may experience auditory and visual hallucinations. *Nursing Process:* Collecting data *Client Need:* Psychosocial integrity
100.	②	The roast beef and chocolate pudding provide a high amount of protein and more calories than the third menu which contains protein in the beefburger, but lower calories in the rest of the meal. *Nursing Process:* Implementing *Client Need:* Health promotion/maintenance
101.	①	Rest is of prime importance to reduce the workload of the heart and to allow the body to heal itself. Although fluids and social interaction are also important, nursing care should be planned around providing undisturbed periods of rest. *Nursing Process:* Planning *Client Need:* Physiological integrity

Item #	Correct Answer	Rationale
102.	②	Diabetes mellitus can be controlled not cured. Insulin and other management techniques for the disorder are regulated by the physician. Any other illness upsets the carbohydrate utilization by the body and necessitates immediate action by the physician to keep the diabetes under control. *Nursing Process:* Implementing *Client Need:* Health promotion/maintenance
103.	②	A dilation and curettage dilates the cervix and scrapes the internal lining of the uterus. Vaginal bleeding must be monitored to assess for the possible complication of postoperative hemorrhage. *Nursing Process:* Collecting data *Client Need:* Physiological integrity
104.	④	The goal of the surgical prep is to reduce the number of bacteria present in order to reduce the chance of infection. *Nursing Process:* Implementing *Client Need:* Safe, effective care environment
105.	①	The flow of oxygen and humidity will affect the reading of an oral temperature. *Nursing Process:* Planning *Client Need:* Physiological integrity
106.	③	The oil retention enema lubricates the rectum and softens the stool. The cleansing enema stimulates peristalsis through irritation of the colon and rectum. To achieve maximum results, the lubrication and softening should be done first so that peristalsis initiated by the enema can be effective in expelling the stool. *Nursing Process:* Implementing *Client Need:* Physiological integrity
107.	①	Providing external support to the chest wound by holding a pillow over it will lessen the client's pain. *Nursing Process:* Implementing *Client Need:* Physiological integrity
108.	④	A newly applied cast may take up to 48 hours to dry completely. The cast will not dry adequately unless it is left uncovered. Attempting to speed up the drying process with heat will cause the plaster to become brittle and powdery. Elevating the extremity on pillows will prevent pressure on the cast from the mattress and assist in reducing any swelling which might occur. *Nursing Process:* Implementing *Client Need:* Physiological integrity
109.	②	Aminophylline relaxes the smooth muscle of the bronchi to relieve bronchospasms. The effect on the client is to relieve dyspnea. *Nursing Process:* Evaluating *Client Need:* Physiological integrity

Item #	Correct Answer	Rationale
110.	③	Fowler's position causes organs in the abdominal cavity to fall away from the diaphragm by gravity thus giving the lungs more room to expand. *Nursing Process:* Implementing *Client Need:* Physiological integrity
111.	③	Since the bladder lies in the anterior pelvic cavity, it should be empty prior to the procedure to prevent possible puncture during the procedure or displacement of the uterine cavity and fetus. *Nursing Process:* Implementing *Client Need:* Safe, effective care environment
112.	③	A full bladder displaces and elevates the post-gravid uterus. The firmness found indicates this is not a bleeding problem. The client needs to void for the uterus to descend. *Nursing Process:* Implementing *Client Need:* Health promotion/maintenance
113.	④	A planned exercise program can greatly benefit the person with diabetes. Insulin does not need to be refrigerated, but extremes of temperature are undesirable. Insulin should be taken everyday, even if the person is ill. *Nursing Process:* Evaluation *Client Need:* Health promotion/maintenance
114.	②	As much skin surface as possible should be exposed to light to aid in photodecomposition of the bilirubin. The infant is removed during feeding, but feedings do not need to be held. The infants' eyes must be covered to protect the retina from damage. Temperature should be monitored at least every four hours. *Nursing Process:* Implementing *Client Need:* Health promotion/maintenance
115.	②	Thiazide diuretics deplete potassium. Apricots have the most potassium of the foods listed. *Nursing Process:* Implementing *Client Need:* Health promotion/maintenance
116.	①	Temperature is affected by too many other variables and is not as accurate as pulse. A comparison of extremities gives the degree of occlusion in the affected extremity. *Nursing Process:* Collecting data *Client Need:* Physiological integrity
117.	②	Weight bearing should be on the hands and arms not the axillae. *Nursing Process:* Evaluating *Client Need:* Physiological integrity
118.	④	Urea nitrogen, a by-product of protein metabolism, cannot be excreted by impaired kidneys, thus protein will be restricted. *Nursing Process:* Collecting data *Client Need:* Physiological intergrity

Item #	Correct Answer	Rationale
119.	④	Urinary retention may complicate the procedure due to edema of the urethra. The client will complain of abdominal discomfort. *Nursing Process:* Collecting data *Client Need:* Physiological integrity
120.	④	The collection system should be maintained below the level of the client's chest to prevent backflow of fluid and air into the pleural cavity. *Nursing Process:* Implementing *Client Need:* Physiological integrity

Answers, Part II

Item #	Correct Answer	Rationale
121.	①	Milk is an important source of the whole proteins, and vitamin D is essential for fetal development and maternal health. It is necessary to determine a food allergy to milk or milk products and then recommend alternate sources of the nutrients contained in milk. *Nursing Process:* Collecting data *Client Need:* Health promotion/maintenance
122.	②	Moderation is the key to all activity during pregnancy. *Nursing Process:* Implementing *Client Need:* Health promotion/maintenance
123.	①	Placing the areola (dark area) as well as the nipple in the baby's mouth aids in adequately compressing the milk ducts underneath the pigmented skin. Also, this placement decreases stress on the nipple leading to cracks and soreness. *Nursing Process:* Implementing *Client Need:* Health promotion/maintenance
124.	④	By remaining with Ms. Lasher, the nurse demonstrates empathy and concern for the client. Her supportive presence may encourage Ms. Lasher to verbalize further and better understand her feelings. *Nursing Process:* Implementing *Client Need:* Psychosocial integrity
125.	③	During lactation a mother needs additional calcium and protein in her diet. Milk production places great demand on the mother's resources of both these nutrients. *Nursing Process:* Implementing *Client Need:* Health promotion/maintenance
126.	②	Increased secretion of thyroxin results in an increased metabolic rate which produces insomnia and palpitations. *Nursing Process:* Collecting data *Client Need:* Physiological integrity
127.	④	The protein bound iodine and the T-3 uptake tests are blood studies. The radioactive iodine uptake shows the percentage of radioactive iodine ingested orally stored in the thyroid gland. No special preparation is needed for any of the examinations, however ingesting iodine in the form of iodized salt or drugs may alter the results of the tests. *Nursing Process:* Implementing *Client Need:* Safe, effective care environment
128.	②	In hyperthyroidism, metabolic demand is increased and the body needs readily available energy provided by carbohydrates. The high-calorie, high-carbohydrate, high-vitamin diet helps to prevent liver damage from the depletion of glycogen and vitamin stores. *Nursing Process:* Implementing *Client Need:* Health promotion/maintenance

Item #	Correct Answer	Rationale
129.	③	Iodine will cause nausea and vomiting and will stain the teeth, therefore it is diluted in fruit juice, water, or milk and taken through a straw. *Nursing Process:* Evaluating *Client Need:* Health promotion/maintenance
130.	①	Due to the increased metabolic rate, the client complains of being warm, perspires freely, and is sensitive to heat. *Nursing Process:* Planning *Client Need:* Physiological integrity
131.	②	The supported Fowler's position, with the head of the bed elevated and the knees also elevated, is the best way to maintain a patent airway, decrease the possibility of hemorrhage and rupture of sutures, and maintain client comfort. *Nursing Process:* Implementing *Client Need:* Physiological integrity
132.	②	Steve's pain results from clumping of erythrocytes. This condition results in occlusion of capillaries which decreases oxygen to the cells. The mother has a right to know about her child's disease and treatment. The nurse can best explain Steve's complaints in terms his mother will understand. *Nursing Process:* Implementing *Client Need:* Physiological integrity
133.	①	Steve, at age 8, may be scared and uncertain of what will happen during his hospitalization. Spending time with him when physical care is not being given will show Steve that the nurse's interest is not only in his disease and will give him the opportunity to discuss his fears and concerns. *Nursing Process:* Planning *Client Need:* Health promotion/maintenance
134.	②	At this time there is no cure for sickle cell anemia and the course of the disease varies for each client. It is a chronic disease with crises occurring throughout the client's lifetime at different intervals. It is not considered to be arrested regardless of the time between crises or the age of the client. *Nursing Process:* Evaluating *Client Need:* Physiological integrity
135.	③	Eight-year-olds show a definite preference for group play with children their own age of both sexes. They can structure their own activities and have outgrown the imaginary playmate stage. *Nursing Process:* Planning *Client Need:* Health promotion/maintenance
136.	④	Whenever a change of location is anticipated, the client and the client's family need to know the type and location of medical care facilities available should a sickle cell crisis occur. *Nursing Process:* Planning *Client Need:* Health promotion/maintenance

Item #	Correct Answer	Rationale

137. ② A rash or urticaria is a common symptom of an antibiotic drug reaction. Other symptoms are hypotension, vomiting, diarrhea, respiratory distress and, most seriously, anaphylaxis.
Nursing Process: Collecting data
Client Need: Physiological integrity

138. ① Children, as well as adults, may require analgesia following surgery. However, when children are medicated the dosage is smaller and needs to be calculated according to the child's individual body weight.
Nursing Process: Planning
Client Need: Physiological integrity

139. ④ A 12-year-old is entering puberty and may be self-conscious about secondary sexual characteristics that are developing. Therefore, the nurse needs to be careful to insure privacy.
Nursing Process: Planning
Client Need: Health promotion/maintenance

140. ③ Bed rest will conserve energy and allow the body to use its resources to combat infection.
Nursing Process: Implementing
Client Need: Health promotion/maintenance

141. ④ Use of aseptic technique in collecting Ms. Hale's urine lowers the possibility of contamination with organisms from other sources. Culturing the specimen requires growing the organism, and sensitivity identifies antibiotics the organism is sensitive to.
Nursing Process: Implementing
Client Need: Safe, effective care environment

142. ① As the kidney becomes inflamed and the blood vessels congested, the urine may contain blood. Mucous and pus from the infection may also be seen. The mucous and pus cause the urine to be cloudy. Since these are observations that may be seen in a client with pyelonephritis, they must be recorded and reported.
Nursing Process: Collecting data
Client Need: Safe, effective care environment

143. ① Eggs contain approximately 1.2 mg. of iron per egg; none of the foods in the other answers contain an appreciable amount of iron.
Nursing Process: Evaluating
Client Need: Health promotion/maintenance

144. ③ The nurse needs to find the underlying reason for Ms. Stone's expression of fear about childbirth. Three of the responses dismiss Ms. Stone's fears and cut off any further discussion. The third response allows the nurse to find out more about Ms. Stone's anxiety.
Nursing Process: Implementing
Client Need: Psychosocial integrity

Item #	Correct Answer	Rationale
145.	①	By assessing the consistency of Ms. Stone's uterine fundus the nurse may be able to take steps to control the bleeding. If the fundus is not well contracted, fundal massage may stimulate contraction and reduce bleeding. The nurse may then implement other actions. While all the answers are correct, the best action to take first is number one. *Nursing Process:* Implementing *Client Need:* Health promotion/maintenance
146.	①	Before proceeding with health teaching it is always best to assess the client's level of knowledge on the subject. By finding out what Ms. Stone knows about available services, the nurse can assist her in making a decision about further counseling. *Nursing Process:* Collecting data *Client Need:* Health promotion/maintenance
147.	②	By giving the client the cue that discussion of feelings is healthy, the nurse encourages her to talk about her reaction to her pregnancy. It also gives recognition to the importance of these feelings. *Nursing Process:* Implementing *Client Need:* Psychosocial integrity
148.	④	The nurse understands that women over 35 and women who have had five or more pregnancies are considered high-risk mothers. *Nursing Process:* Implementing *Client Need:* Health promotion/maintenance
149.	④	Breast-feeding is based on supply and demand. Therefore, the more the baby sucks, the more milk is produced. The sucking and emptying of the breast stimulates release of hormones which signal milk production. *Nursing Process:* Implementing *Client Need:* Health promotion/maintenance
150.	③	Oral contraceptives are approximately 99% effective when taken as directed. The factors mentioned in the other answers do not influence the effectiveness of oral contraceptives. *Nursing Process:* Evaluating *Client Need:* Health promotion/maintenance
151.	②	Since itching may be intense in the child with eczema, Linda will try to scratch herself. Keeping her fingernails cut short will lessen the chance of secondary infection developing. *Nursing Process:* Implementing *Client Need:* Health promotion/maintenance
152.	②	A normal 3-month-old will respond with a smile when spoken to. *Nursing Process:* Collecting data *Client Need:* Health promotion/maintenance

Item #	Correct Answer	Rationale
153.	①	Linda's elbow restraints can be removed when she is being held. When an adult is holding her, she is restrained naturally. She can move freely and have the advantage of being touched, while still being prevented from scratching the areas of eczema. *Nursing Process:* Implementing *Client Need:* Safe, effective care environment
154.	②	Eczema is considered to be essentially an allergic response and one of the symptoms is itching that may be reduced with antihistamines. *Nursing Process:* Evaluating *Client Need:* Physiological integrity
155.	③	If the tube formed by a sac of peritoneum does not atrophy after the descent of the testis in utero, the intestine may descend into that sac and produce an inguinal hernia. The hernia is a visible mass in the groin. *Nursing Process:* Collecting data *Client Need:* Physiological integrity
156.	①	At 20 months, children are frequently attached to objects. The object becomes extremely important, particularly if the child is frightened. The comment that best indicates the nurse's understanding of such an attachment is, "It looks as if that's Bobby's favorite blanket. It is all right for him to keep it with him." *Nursing Process:* Implementing *Client Need:* Health promotion/maintenance
157.	②	A child of 20 months cannot be expected to remain still during a painful procedure. To insure a quick, successful venipuncture, it is important that the nurse hold Bobby's arm firmly in position. *Nursing Process:* Implementing *Client Need:* Safe, effective care environment
158.	③	It is normal for Bobby to cry when his mother leaves. Bobby's mother needs to be reassured that someone will be with her child to comfort him. "I'll stay here with Bobby and try to comfort him," is the best response. *Nursing Process:* Implementing *Client Need:* Psychosocial integrity
159.	①	Bobby will be unhappy and thirsty when he cannot drink. While mouthwash and an explanation might work well for an adult or older child, Bobby will not understand and he may swallow the mouthwash. Ice cannot be given to anyone who is to have nothing by mouth. Taking Bobby for a walk is the most appropriate intervention because distraction is an effective technique for dealing with a 20-month-old. *Nursing Process:* Planning *Client Need:* Physiological integrity

Item #	Correct Answer	Rationale
160.	③	Cheese is a good milk substitute. It contains large amounts of calcium and is not as high in calories as cream. Citrus juices and root vegetables do not offer the protein of milk. *Nursing Process:* Implementing *Client Need:* Health promotion/maintenance
161.	③	Every effort should be made to avoid further aggravation of Anna's respiratory distress. The nurse should postpone taking respirations until the child becomes quiet. *Nursing Process:* Evaluating *Client Need:* Physiological integrity
162.	④	The nurse should explain to Ms. Garcia that the function of the croup tent is to generate high humidity to aid in thinning respiratory secretions. The dampness of Anna's clothing is due to condensation and is nothing to be alarmed about. *Nursing Process:* Implementing *Client Need:* Physiological integrity
163.	①	One of the safety rules of oxygen administration is to "flush" enclosed units with oxygen before placing the client inside them. *Nursing Process:* Implementing *Client Need:* Safe, effective care environment
164.	④	The 2-year-old child engages in parallel play, that is, playing alongside but not actually with other children. *Nursing Process:* Collecting data *Client Need:* Health promotion/maintenance
165.	②	The client is showing symptoms of impaired circulation. Nothing should be done to further impede her circulation, and the weight of the bed linen could be a source of pressure. *Nursing Process:* Implementing *Client Need:* Physiological integrity
166.	③	Sterile technique reduces the risk of introducing additional microorganisms into the wound. Clients with diabetes heal poorly and their treatment should include prevention of infection. *Nursing Process:* Implementing *Client Need:* Safe, effective care environment
167.	③	Polydipsia and polyuria are symptoms of diabetes mellitus. *Nursing Process:* Collecting data *Client Need:* Physiological integrity
168.	③	NPH insulin is an intermediate acting insulin with a peak action of six to eight hours. During peak action time, maximum insulin effect is expected to occur. To prevent an insulin reaction, proper food supplements must be given. *Nursing Process:* Implementing *Client Need:* Health promotion/maintenance

Item #	Correct Answer	Rationale

169. ① Ms. Young has insulin-dependent diabetes mellitus so the use of oral hypoglycemic drugs is contraindicated.
Nursing Process: Implementing
Client Need: Health promotion/maintenance

170. ① Nicotine is a vasoconstrictor and contributes to progressive peripheral vascular disease.
Nursing Process: Implementing
Client Need: Health promotion/maintenance

171. ② To avoid injury to the toes, the nurse should cut her toe nails straight across. Even slight abrasions or scratches can lead to serious problems for clients with diabetes because of their impaired circulation.
Nursing Process: Planning
Client Need: Physiological integrity

172. ① The onset of diabetic ketoacidosis is gradual, the specific cause being lack of insulin and eventual accumulation of glucose and waste products from excessive fat and protein metabolism. Ms. Young should be instructed to recognize thirst and drowsiness as symptoms of diabetic ketoacidosis.
Nursing Process: Planning
Client Need: Health promotion/maintenance

173. ② Since Ms. Varnick has bright red vaginal bleeding, the nurse needs to assess her for symptoms of hemorrhage. By taking her blood pressure and pulse rate first, a baseline can be established and these signs can be established and evaluated.
Nursing Process: Collecting data
Client Need: Physiological integrity

174. ① Spinal anesthesia may cause a headache due to leakage of cerebrospinal fluid (CSF) through the hole in the dura. To prevent this, the client should remain flat in bed (preferably prone) to slow down leakage of CSF. The other measures are important and should be included but are not a priority.
Nursing Process: Planning
Client Need: Physiological integrity

175. ③ The nurse has recognized the symptoms of hemorrhage and wisely checked the abdominal dressings. The nurse needs to be aware that the client may be hemorrhaging via the vagina and should also check the perineal pad and assess the amount of lochia.
Nursing Process: Implementing
Client Need: Physiological integrity

176. ④ Bright red moderate lochia on the fourth day postpartum is a deviation from normal. Lochia should be pink, serous, and blood tinged from day 4 until day 7 to 10. The correct answer is to report this finding to the registered nurse in charge for further assessment.
Nursing Process: Implementing
Client Need: Safe, effective care environment

Item #	Correct Answer	Rationale
177.	①	The virus causing herpes zoster is similar to the causative agent of chickenpox. *Nursing Process:* Collecting data *Client Need:* Safe, effective care environment
178.	④	The pain of herpes zoster is a burning one. Cool compresses constrict the circulation and slow nerve impulses thus relieving the itching and burning pain. *Nursing Process:* Planning *Client Need:* Physiological integrity
179.	②	The pain usually persists for up to a month, but could indicate a neuralgic pain called postherpetic neuralgia which persists long after the lesions have subsided. *Nursing Process:* Implementing *Client Need:* Health promotion/maintenance
180.	③	Having conflicts between dependence and independence is a normal characteristic of adolescents moving toward adulthood. These conflicts represent a search for identity. *Nursing Process:* Collecting data *Client Need:* Health promotion/maintenance
181.	④	The ultimate source of all vitamin A is plants, especially those with carotene. Carrots and sweet potatoes are the only foods listed that have carotene. *Nursing Process:* Implementing *Client Need:* Health promotion/maintenance
182.	②	Glaucoma is caused by changes in the anterior chamber of the eye, which prevent normal outflow of aqueous humor and cause increased intraocular pressure. Continued pressure causes damage to the optic nerve and visual loss. If the disease is not treated blindness will occur. *Nursing Process:* Implementing *Client Need:* Health promotion/maintenance
183.	③	A comatose client, unable to move independently, can develop many side effects including pneumonia and decubitus ulcers. Turning the client from side to side at regular intervals will distribute the pressure among many points, decreasing the possibility of decubitus ulcer formation. These position changes will also help drain secretions from the lungs. *Nursing Process:* Planning *Client Need:* Physiological integrity
184.	④	A liver biopsy is an invasive technique involving the use of a special biopsy needle. Hemorrhage is a complication that will appear in the first hours following this procedure. *Nursing Process:* Collecting data *Client Need:* Physiological integrity

Item #	Correct Answer	Rationale
185.	②	Introduction of colostomy irrigation fluid under high pressure can lead to perforation of the intestines. Since the irrigation fluid is introduced using a simple pressure principle, the nurse should understand that the pressure of the fluid will be increased the higher the fluid container is held above the client. Pressure can be reduced by placing the irrigation fluid container near the level of the client's abdomen. *Nursing Process:* Implementing *Client Need:* Health promotion/maintenance
186.	④	Preeclampsia is the syndrome of hypertension with proteinuria and edema. The nurse recognizes persistent headaches and blurred vision as signs of elevated blood pressure. *Nursing Process:* Collecting data *Client Need:* Health promotion/maintenance
187.	②	It is important to change the baby's position at regular intervals to prevent the development of pressure sores on the baby's head. The feeding schedule should be flexible, not established to accommodate diagnostic procedures. Head circumference should be measured daily. *Nursing Process:* Planning *Client Need:* Physiological integrity
188.	②	Holding the infant in an upright position during feeding facilitates swallowing, burping, and retention of formula. It also prevents aspiration or vomiting. *Nursing Process:* Implementing *Client Need:* Physiological integrity
189.	①	Small, frequent feedings will prevent discomfort. The nurse should instruct the boy about smaller portions to insure his understanding and cooperation. *Nursing Process:* Evaluating *Client Need:* Physiological integrity
190.	④	Sending the man to the emergency room is the most appropriate action. Early detection and treatment of an eye injury may prevent permanent damage and disability. The nurse should not treat the man on the unit. *Nursing Process:* Implementing *Client Need:* Physiological integrity
191.	①	Rehabilitation is necessary after a modified radical mastectomy because underlying tissues are removed. The aim of rehabilitation is to restore use of the affected arm as soon as possible to prevent contractures and muscle shortening, maintain muscle tone, and improve circulation in the arm. *Nursing Process:* Implementing *Client Need:* Health promotion/maintenance

Item #	Correct Answer	Rationale

192.   ①   Trauma to the mucous membranes should be minimized during suctioning. Care should be taken during insertion of the cather and the suction should be maintained only intermittently for no longer than 10 to 15 seconds at a time. Client should be hyperoxygenated before and after the procedure.
Nursing Process: Implementing
Client Need: Physiological integrity

193.   ②   Antabuse reacts within the body when alcohol is ingested, causing the client to become violently ill. Alcohol is present in many ingested substances, i.e., foods, over the counter medication, etc. The body reacts to this hidden alcohol the same as if the client had ingested alcohol alone.
Nursing Process: Evaluating
Client Need: Physiological integrity

194.   ②   The primary purpose for the upright position is to prevent reflux of the feeding back through the cardiac sphincter. With the client in an upright position, the feeding flows by gravity into the pyloric portion of the stomach. Regurgitation and the resulting aspiration are common complications of the procedure. This can be minimized by keeping the client in an upright position for approximately one hour after feeding.
Nursing Process: Implementing
Client Need: Physiological integrity

195.   ③   After anesthesia and abdominal surgery, peristalsis is temporarily halted and usually does not return for approximately 36 to 48 hours. Absence of bowel sounds 12 hours after surgery would be normal and should just be recorded on the client's chart.
Nursing Process: Evaluating
Client Need: Physiological integrity

196.   ④   To keep the donor site soft and scarring at a minimum, lotion or lanolin cream should be rubbed in several times a day.
Nursing Process: Implementing
Client Need: Health promotion/maintenance

197.   ④   Food is exchangeable on the ADA food exchange lists. Each item on a specific list is equal in nutritional value. Similar amounts are interchangeable with one another. If the client dislikes a certain food, another of equal value is substituted from that list.
Nursing Process: Implementing
Client Need: Health promotion/maintenance

198.   ①   Sputum laden tissues should be confined to a closed area which can be disposed of into institutional incinerators or burned. Proper handling of sputum prevents the organisms from becoming airborne. Distractor number 4 is not appropriate because no teaching is involved.
Nursing Process: Implementing
Client Need: Safe, effective care environment

Item #	Correct Answer	Rationale
199.	②	An enteric coated tablet is so designed to pass through the stomach and slowly be dissolved and absorbed through the intestinal tract. Crushing the tablet removes this safeguard. Further instructions must be obtained about how to best administer this medication. *Nursing Process:* Evaluating *Client Need:* Physiological integrity
200.	③	The walker and the weaker leg are moved first. The body weight is borne by the stronger leg. The stronger leg is moved into the walker while the weight is borne by the arms on the walker and the weak leg. *Nursing Process:* Evaluating *Client Need:* Physiological integrity
201.	②	Positioning the client on his or her side promotes drainage of saliva and prevents the tongue from falling back to obstruct the airway. Sleep is normal due to the expending of great amounts of energy during the seizure. *Nursing Process:* Implementing *Client Need:* Physiological integrity
202.	②	Stupor is classified as having inappropriate responses with the client confused or delirious and very difficult to arouse. There is some voluntary movement and reflex withdrawal to strong stimuli. *Nursing Process:* Evaluating *Client Need:* Physiological integrity
203.	②	While relief of symptoms is the purpose of the procedure, this does not give information regarding reaction during the procedure. Since vasodilation occurs, monitoring cardiac status by checking pulse and skin color is the best indicator of response. *Nursing Process:* Evaluating *Client Need:* Physiological integrity
204.	③	In a child, the ear canal is straightened by pulling the ear lobe gently down and back. This facilitates the medication reaching the complete ear canal and ear drum. Cooperation with the parents is preferred, but not essential. The child only needs to stay on the side for two to three minutes. *Nursing Process:* Implementing *Client Need:* Physiological integrity
205.	①	A stable environment is crucial in minimizing confusion due to memory loss. Focusing on present events, including the client in all activities, and introducing the client to multiple people only enhance confusion as the client has difficulty grasping current activities and faces. *Nursing Process:* Planning *Client Need:* Psychosocial integrity

Item #	Correct Answer	Rationale
206.	③	$0.05 \text{ mg} = 0.08 \text{ mg}$ $1 \text{ cc} \quad x$ $0.05 \text{ mg } x = 0.08 \text{ mg/cc}$ $x = 1.6 \text{ cc}$ *Nursing Process:* Implementing *Client Need:* Physiological integrity
207.	①	Unconsciousness may follow a seizure and the client may be unable to clear nasal and pharyngeal secretions, thus suction equipment and oxygen should be available. *Nursing Process:* Planning *Client Need:* Physiological integrity
208.	③	The child with a chronic illness is at risk for overprotection particularly if the condition is perceived as causing the child to be vulnerable. Emotional and physical development can be stunted if overprotection occurs. *Nursing Process:* Evaluating *Client Need:* Health promotion/maintenance
209.	①	The anatomical position of the eustachian tube in children predisposes organisms from the nasopharynx to travel up the tube and enter the middle ear. *Nursing Process:* Implementing *Client Need:* Health promotion/maintenance
210.	③	Expectorants are used to improve the removal of secretions by thinning mucus and decreasing its viscosity. *Nursing Process:* Evaluating *Client Need:* Physiological integrity
211.	②	The intervertebral disc thins during the aging process diminishing height by 1 to 2 inches by the eigth decade. *Nursing Process:* Collecting data *Client Need:* Health promotion/maintenance
212.	④	Movement of joints is recommended to prevent contractures and to maintain functioning. *Nursing Process:* Implementing *Client Need:* Health promotion/maintenance
213.	③	Hepatitis A is spread predominantly through the fecal-oral route, thus enteric precautions should be followed. *Nursing Process:* Planning *Client Need:* Safe, effective care environment
214.	③	There is a rare chance of transmitting the disease to a transfusion recipient. *Nursing Process:* Evaluating *Client Need:* Safe, effective care environment

Item #	Correct Answer	Rationale

215.   ③

Any movement of the affected extremity increases the potential for release of a thrombus which could travel through the circulatory system to a vital structure.
Nursing Process: Implementing
Client Need: Health promotion/maintenance

216.   ②

Heparin prevents the activation of clotting factor IX and inhibits the action of thrombin in forming fibrin threads. Its effect can be determined by measuring the Lee-White clotting time, the activated partial thromboplastin time, or the partial thromboplastin time.
Nursing Process: Evaluating
Client Need: Physiological integrity

217.   ④

The small water droplets in humidified air act as an expectorant to loosen dry secretions in the bronchi and trachea.
Nursing Process: Implementing
Client Need: Safe, effective care environment

218.   ③

Spacing activities diminishes the amount of oxygen needed at any one time and allows the oxygen reserves to be built up during periods of rest.
Nursing Process: Planning
Client Need: Physiological integrity

219.   ②

A high fluid intake will dilute urine and decrease mucosal irritation. The increase in urine volume will also facilitate maintenance of catheter patency. Drinking cranberry juice will not decrease the risk of infection.
Nursing Process: Implementing
Client Need: Health promotion/maintenance

220.   ②

A stone may be passed at any time, thus all urine of a client with renal calculus should be strained.
Nursing Process: Implementing
Client Need: Safe, effective care environment

221.   ④

Puerperal infection is identified when a client exhibits an oral temperature of 100.4°F (38.0°C) occurring on any postpartum day starting two days after delivery.
Nursing Process: Collecting data
Client Need: Safe, effective care environment

222.   ④

Increased diastolic pressure which is due to increased peripheral resistance is the greatest indicator of hypertension.
Nursing Process: Evaluating
Client Need: Physiological integrity

223.   ④

It is important for the parents to keep a record of the child's immunizations and to know the infant may be irritable, however, that is not the most important point to stress. Parents should seek immediate help if the child becomes very lethargic, has persistent screaming episodes, high fever, or seizures.
Nursing Process: Implementing
Client Need: Health promotion/maintenance

Item #	Correct Answer	Rationale
224.	④	A positive reaction to a tuberculosis skin test indicates that a person has been infected at some time in his or her life to the tubercle bacillus. It does not indicate whether the infection is currently active or inactive. *Nursing Process:* Evaluating *Client Need:* Health promotion/maintenance
225.	②	The best solution to the immediate problem is to separate the roommates. Once they have cooled off, talking with them may help to ease the conflict and allow them to work out their problems. *Nursing Process:* Implementing *Client Need:* Safe, effective care environment
226.	②	A child's head should not be hyperextended during CPR because the trachea is soft and hyperextension my compress it. Breathing into the nose and mouth simultaneously is only appropriate in infants under 1 year of age. *Nursing Process:* Implementing *Client Need:* Physiological integrity
227.	④	The ointment should be applied using the specially designed dose-determining applicator supplied with the medication. The ointment should be placed onto the desired area of skin. Spread the ointment over at least a 2 X 3-inch area in a thin uniform layer using the applicator. Cover the area with plastic wrap, which can be held in place by adhesive tape. Do not touch the ointment with fingertips. *Nursing Process:* Implementing *Client Need:* Physiological integrity
228.	②	The most appropriate approach is to ask the client's wife how she would like to help. If she doesn't feel comfortable helping, this allows her to say so. If she does want to help, she can assist with simple care measures. *Nursing Process:* Implementing *Client Need:* Health promotion/maintenance
229.	③	This response acknowledges the nursing assistant's legitimate feelings of hostility toward the parents. Before the nurse can begin helping to develop a therapeutic staff attitude toward the parents, she should encourage those feelings to be expressed to her. By doing so, the nursing assistant may be able to deal more effectively with the parents. *Nursing Process:* Implementing *Client Need:* Safe, effective care environment
230.	④	Patients with chronic pain may require large doses of narcotics to keep them comfortable. This dosage is very appropriate and may become much higher in the future if the client's condition warrants. *Nursing Process:* Evaluating *Client Need:* Physiological integrity

Item #	Correct Answer	Rationale
231.	③	Information in a client's record should be accurate, concise, thorough, current, and organized. Entry number 3 is the only one that has the time listed. This is essential to assure that the charting is current. *Nursing Process:* Collecting data *Client Need:* Safe, effective care environment
232.	④	Gastrointestinal irritation is the most common symptom after plant ingestion. Inducing vomiting attempts to remove the toxin before it is absorbed. Saving the vomitus permits analysis of the contents. *Nursing Process:* Implementation *Client Need:* Physiological integrity
233.	②	The best position is the left side-lying Sims' position with the right knee flexed. This allows the medication to be inserted into the natural curve of the sigmird colon and rectum. Number 1 is acceptable, but not the best. *Nursing Process:* Implementing *Client Need:* Physiological integrity
234.	①	Lay people are no longer taught two-rescuer CPR. If the rescuer tires, another trained person may take over. *Nursing Process:* Implementing *Client Need:* Physiological integrity
235.	③	Toilet isolation is important to prevent spread and/or reinfection. The best way to handle the problem is to discuss it with the client and the client's friend. The friend must know the precautions to take so as not to become infected. Recording it in the nurse's note and telling the nurse in charge can be done later. *Nursing Process:* Implementing *Client Need:* Safe, effective care environment
236.	②	Combining exercise with dieting is essential. In trying to determine an exercise program that the client will comply with, the nurse should start with finding out what the client enjoys. *Nursing Process:* Collecting data *Client Need:* Health promotion/maintenance
237.	①	The prosthesis should be stored in water in a plastic storage case labeled with the client's name and placed in the bedside stand. The water maintains the condition of prosthesis and labelling prevents loss. Some clients may use contact lens soaking solution in the container. Use of sterile supplies is not necessary. *Nursing Process:* Implementing *Client Need:* Physiological integrity
238.	②	The client will be taken to an area of the hospital designated for external radiation therapy treatments. The client will not be radioactive, so there is no need to restrict visitors or place the client in isolation. *Nursing Process:* Evaluating *Client Need:* Physiological integrity

Item #	Correct Answer	Rationale

239.   ④   Following a cardiac catheterization, the blood pressure and pulse should be taken every 15 minutes for the first hour. In addition, the pulses, color, warmth, and sensation of the extremity distal to the insertion site should be checked every 15 minutes for the first hour also. Since the femoral artery was used, the head of the bed should not be elevated. Coughing is not important because general anesthesia was not used.
Nursing Process: Collecting data
Client Need: Safe, effective care environment

240.   ①   The nurse should wash her hands first before beginning any procedure. The sterile field should be prepared and the soiled dressing removed before sterile gloves are donned.
Nursing Process: Implementing
Client Need: Physiological integrity

Appendix

Administration of Examination Committee Testing Dates

NCLEX for *Registered Nurse* Licensure

1990: February 6-7 and July 11-12
1991: February 5-6 and July 9-10
1992: February 5-6 and July 8-9
1993: February 3-4 and July 7-8
1994: February 2-3 and July 13-14
1995: February 8-9 and July 12-13
1996: February 6-7 and July 9-10
1997: February 4-5 and July 15-16
1998: February 3-4 and July 14-15
1999: February 2-3 and July 13-14

NCLEX for *Practical Nurse* Licensure

1990: April 18 and October 16
1991: April 16 and October 16
1992: April 15 and October 21
1993: April 14 and October 13
1994: April 13 and October 12
1995: April 12 and October 24
1996: April 17 and October 16
1997: April 16 and October 9
1998: April 7 and October 20
1999: April 14 and October 13

State and Territorial Boards of Nursing and Practical Nursing

National Council of State Boards of Nursing, Inc.

ALABAMA
Executive Officer
Alabama Board of Nursing
RSA Plaza, Suite 250
770 Washington Avenue
Montgomery, Alabama 36130
Tel: (205) 242-4060
Fax: (205) 242-4360

ALASKA
Executive Secretary
Alaska Board of Nursing
Department of Commerce and Economic
    Development
Division of Occupational Licensing
3601 C Street, Suite 722
Anchorage, Alaska 99503
Tel: (907) 561-2878
Fax: (907) 562-5781

AMERICAN SAMOA
Executive Secretary
American Samoa Health Service Regulatory
    Board
LBJ Tropical Medical Center
Pago Pago, American Samoa 96799
Tel: (684) 633-1222 Ext. 206
Telex No.: #782-573-LBJ TMC
Fax: (684) 633-1869

ARIZONA
Executive Director
Arizona State Board of Nursing
2001 West Camelback Road, Suite 350
Phoenix, Arizona 85015
Tel: (602) 255-5092
Fax: (602) 255-5130

ARKANSAS
Executive Director
Arkansas State Board of Nursing
University Tower Building, Suite 800
1123 South University
Little Rock, Arkansas 72204
Tel: (501) 686-2700
Fax: (501) 686-2714

CALIFORNIA
Executive Officer
California Board of Registered Nursing
400 R Street, Suite 4030
Sacramento, California 95814
Tel: (916) 322-3350
Fax: (916) 327-4402

Executive Officer
California Board of Vocational Nurse and
    Psychiatric Technician Examiners
1414 K Street, Suite 103
Sacramento, California 95814
Tel: (916) 445-0793
Fax: (916) 327-4408

COLORADO
Program Administrator
Colorado Board of Nursing
1560 Broadway, Suite 670
Denver, Colorado 80202
Tel: (303) 894-2430
Fax: (303) 894-2821

CONNECTICUT
Executive Officer
Connecticut Board of Examiners for Nursing
150 Washington Street
Hartford, Connecticut 06106
Tel: (203) 566-1041
Fax: (203) 566-8401

DELAWARE
Executive Director
Delaware Board of Nursing
Margaret O'Neill Building
P.O. Box 1401
Dover, Delaware 19903
Tel: (302) 739-4522
Fax: (302) 739-6148

DISTRICT OF COLUMBIA
District of Columbia Board of Nursing
614 H Street, N.W.
Washington, D.C. 20001
Tel: (202) 727-7468
Fax: (202) 727-8030

FLORIDA
Executive Director
Florida Board of Nursing
111 Coastline Drive, East, Suite 510
Jacksonville, Florida 32202
Tel: (904) 359-6331

GEORGIA
Executive Director
Georgia Board of Licensed Practical Nurses
166 Pryor Street, S.W.
Atlanta, Georgia 30303
Tel: (404) 656-3943
Fax: (404) 651-9532

Executive Director
Georgia State Board of Licensed Practical
  Nurses
166 Pryor Street, S.W.
Atlanta, Georgia 30303
Tel: (404) 656-3921
Fax: (404) 656-9532

GUAM
Nurse Examiner Administrator
Guam Board of Nurse Examiners
P.O. Box 2816
Agana, Guam 96910
Tel: (671) 734-7295
Fax: (671) 734-2066

HAWAII
Executive Secretary
Hawaii Board of Nursing
P.O. Box 3469
Honolulu, Hawaii 96801
Tel: (808) 586-2695
Fax: (808) 586-2689

IDAHO
Executive Director
Idaho Board of Nursing
280 North 8th Street, Suite 210
Boise, Idaho 83720
Tel: (208) 334-3110

ILLINOIS
Chief Testing Officer
Illinois Department of Professional
  Regulation
320 West Washington Street
Springfield, Illinois 62786
Tel: (217) 785-0800
Fax: (217) 782-7645

Nursing Coordinator
Illinois Department of Professional
  Regulation
159 North Dearborn, 6th Floor
Chicago, Illinois 60601
Tel: (312) 814-4619
Fax: (312) 814-1664

INDIANA

Executive Director
Indiana State Board of Nursing
Health Professions Bureau
402 West Washington Street, Room #041
Indianapolis, Indiana 46204
Tel: (317) 232-2960
Fax: (317) 233-4236

IOWA

Executive Director
Iowa Board of Nursing
State Capitol Complex
1223 East Court Avenue
Des Moines, Iowa 50319
Tel: (515) 281-3255

KANSAS

Executive Administrator
Kansas Board of Nursing
Landon State Office Building
900 SW Jackson, Suite 551 S
Topeka, Kansas 66612-1256
Tel: (913) 296-4068
Fax: (913) 296-6729

KENTUCKY

Executive Director
Kentucky Board of Nursing
4010 Dupont Circle, Suite 430
Louisville, Kentucky 40207
Tel: (502) 897-5143
Fax: (502) 588-3122

LOUISIANA

Executive Director
Louisiana State Board of Nursing
907 Pere Marquette Building
150 Baronne Street
New Orleans, Louisiana 70112
Tel: (504) 568-5464
Fax: (504) 568-5467

Executive Director
Louisiana State Board of Practical Nurse
  Examiners
Tidewater Place
1440 Canal Street, Suite 1722
New Orleans, Louisiana 70112
Tel: (504) 568-6480
Fax: (504) 568-6482

MAINE

Executive Director
Maine State Board of Nursing
State House Station #158
Augusta, Maine 04333-0158
Tel: (207) 624-5275

MARYLAND

Executive Director
Maryland Board of Nursing
4201 Patterson Avenue
Baltimore, Maryland 21215-2299
Tel: (301) 764-4741
Fax: (301) 764-5987

MASSACHUSETTS

Executive Secretary
Massachusetts Board of Registration in
  Nursing
Leverett Saltonstall Building
100 Cambridge Street, Room 1519
Boston, Massachusetts 02202
Tel: (617) 727-9962
Fax: (617) 727-7378

MICHIGAN

Licensing Administrator
Bureau of Occupational and Professional
  Regulation Michigan Department of
  Commerce
Ottawa Towers North
611 West Ottawa
Lansing, Michigan 48933
Tel: (517) 373-1600
Fax: (517) 373-2179

MINNESOTA

Executive Director
Minnesota Board of Nursing
2700 University Avenue, West #108
St. Paul, Minnesota 55114
Tel: (612) 642-0567
Fax: (612) 642-0574

MISSISSIPPI

Executive Director
Mississippi Board of Nursing
239 North Lamar Street, Suite 401
Jackson, Mississippi 39201-1311
Tel: (601) 359-6170
Fax: (601) 359-6185

MISSOURI

Executive Director
Missouri State Board of Nursing
3605 Missouri Boulevard
Jefferson City, Missouri 65109
Tel: (314) 751-0681
Fax: (314) 751-4176

MONTANA

Executive Director
Montana State Board of Nursing
Department of Commerce
Arcade Building, Lower Level
111 North Jackson
Helena, Montana 59620-0407
Tel: (406) 444-4279
Fax: (406) 444-2903

NEBRASKA

Associate Director
Bureau of Examining Boards
Nebraska Department of Health
301 Centennial Mall South
Lincoln, Nebraska 68508
Tel: (402) 471-2115
Fax: (402) 471-0383

NEVADA

Executive Director
Nevada State Board of Nursing
1281 Terminal Way, Suite 116
Reno, Nevada 89502
Tel: (702) 786-2778

NEW HAMPSHIRE

Executive Director
New Hampshire Board of Nursing
Health & Welfare Building
6 Hazen Drive
Concord, New Hampshire 03301-6527
Tel: (603) 271-2323
Fax: (603) 271-3825

NEW JERSEY

Executive Director
New Jersey Board of Nursing
124 Halsey Street, 6th Floor
Newark, New Jersey 07102
Tel: (201) 648-2570
Fax: (201) 648-6061

NEW MEXICO

Executive Director
New Mexico Board of Nursing
4253 Montgomery Boulevard
Suite 130
Albuquerque, New Mexico 87109
Tel: (505) 841-8340

NEW YORK

Executive Secretary
New York State Board for Nursing
State Education Department
Cultural Education Center, Room 9B30
Albany, New York 12230
Tel: (518) 474-3845
Fax: (518) 473-0578

NORTH CAROLINA

Executive Director
North Carolina Board of Nursing
3724 National Drive
Raleigh, North Carolina 27612
Tel: (919) 782-3211
Fax: (919) 781-9461

NORTH DAKOTA

Executive Director
North Dakota Board of Nursing
919 South 7th Street, Suite 504
Bismark, North Dakota 58504-5881
Tel: (701) 224-2974
Fax: (701) 224-4614

NORTHERN MARIANA ISLANDS

Chairperson
Commonwealth Board of Nurse Examiners
Public Health Center
P.O. Box 1458
Saipan, MP 96950
Tel: (670) 234-8950
Ask for Public Health Center
Extension: 2018 or 2019
Telex No.: 783-744
Answer back code: PNESPN744
Fax: (670) 234-8930

OHIO

Executive Director
Ohio Board of Nursing
77 South High Street, 17th Floor
Columbus, Ohio 43266-0316
Tel: (614) 466-3947
Fax: (614) 466-0388

OKLAHOMA

Executive Director
Oklahoma Board of Nurse Registration &
  Nursing Education
2915 North Classen Boulevard
Suite 524
Oklahoma City, Oklahoma 73106
Tel: (405) 525-2076
Fax: (405) 521-6089

OREGON

Executive Director
Oregon State Board of Nursing
800 NE Oregon Street, #25
Portland, Oregon 97232
Tel: (503) 731-4745
Fax: (503) 731-4755

PENNSYLVANIA

Executive Secretary
Pennsylvania State Board of Nursing
Transportation & Safety Building
Commonwealth Avenue & Forester Street
Room 611
Harrisburg, Pennsylvania 17105-2649
Tel: (717) 783-7142
Fax: (717) 787-7769

PUERTO RICO

Director, Examining Boards
Commonwealth of Puerto Rico
Board of Nurse Examiners
Call Box 10200
Santurce, Puerto Rico 00908
Tel: (809) 725-8161

RHODE ISLAND

Executive Director
Rhode Island Board of Nurse Registration &
  Nursing Education
Cannon Health Building
Three Capitol Hill, Room 104
Providence, Rhode Island 02908-5097
Tel: (401) 277-2827
Fax: (401) 277-1272

SOUTH CAROLINA

Executive Director
South Carolina State Board of Nursing
220 Executive Center Drive, Suite 220
Columbia, South Carolina 29210
Tel: (803) 731-1648
Fax: (803) 731-1647

SOUTH DAKOTA

Executive Secretary
South Dakota Board of Nursing
3307 South Lincoln Avenue
Sioux Falls, South Dakota 57105-5224
Tel: (605) 335-4973
Fax: (605) 335-2977

TENNESSEE

Executive Director
Tennessee State Board of Nursing
283 Plus Park Boulevard
Nashville, Tennessee 37247-1010
Tel: (615) 367-6232
Fax: (615) 367-6397

TEXAS

Executive Director
Texas Board of Nurse Examiners
9101 Burnet Road
Austin, Texas 78758
Tel: (512) 835-4880
Fax: (512) 835-8684

Executive Director
Texas Board of Vocational Nurse Examiners
9101 Burnet Road, Suite 105
Austin, Texas 78758
Tel: (512) 835-2071

UTAH
Executive Secretary
Utah State Board of Nursing
Division of Occupational & Professional
  Licensing
Heber M. Wells Building, 4th Floor
160 East 300 South
Salt Lake City, Utah 84111
Tel: (801) 530-6628
Fax: (801) 530-6511

VERMONT
Executive Director
Vermont State Board of Nursing
Redstone Building
26 Terrace Street
Montpelier, Vermont 05602-1106
Tel: (802) 828-2396
Fax: (802) 828-2496

VIRGIN ISLANDS
Executive Secretary
Virgin Islands Board of Nurse Licensure
P.O. Box 4247, Veterans Drive Station
St. Thomas, Virgin Islands 00803
Tel: (809) 776-7397

VIRGINIA
Executive Director
Virginia State Board of Nursing
1601 Rolling Hills Drive
Richmond, Virginia 23229-5005
Tel: (804) 662-9909
Fax: (804) 662-9943

WASHINGTON
Executive Secretary
Washington State Board of Nursing
Department of Health
1300 Quince Street, MSEY-27
Olympia, Washington 98504
Tel: (206) 753-2686
Fax: (206) 586-5935

Executive Secretary
Washington State Board of Practical Nursing
1300 SE Quince Street
P.O. Box 47865
Olympia, Washington 98504-7865
Tel: (206) 753-2807
Fax: (206) 753-1338

WEST VIRGINIA
Executive Secretary
West Virginia Board of Examiners for
  Registered Nurses
922 Quarrier Street
Embleton Building, Suite 309
Charleston, West Virginia 25301-2679
Tel: (304) 558-3596
Fax: (304) 558-3666

Executive Secretary
West Virginia State Board of Examiners for
  Practical Nurses
922 Quarrier Street
Embleton Building, Suite 506
Charleston, West Virginia 25301
Tel: (304) 558-3572
Fax: (304) 345-6948

WISCONSIN
Director
Wisconsin Bureau of Health Service
  Professions
1400 East Washington Avenue
P.O. Box 8935
Madison, Wisconsin 53708-8935
Tel: (608) 266-0257
Fax: (608) 267-0644

WYOMING
Executive Director
Wyoming State Board of Nursing
Barrett Building, 2nd Floor
2301 Central Avenue
Cheyenne, Wyoming 82002
Tel: (307) 777-7601
Fax: (307) 777-6005

EC revises/recommends acceptance of Test Plans

DA adopts new Test Plan

PTS reviews items in pool to determine needs of Test Plan specifications and refers needs to EC

EC selects IW from nominees submitted by Member Boards of Nursing representing approximately ¼th of jurisdictions for RN and ¼th of jurisdictions for PN per year

Selection—Based on qualifications, regional distribution, type of program, and clinical practice. Boards submit nominees on a regularly scheduled basis and may participate more frequently if preferred.

PTS gives confidential directions to IW based on the needs of the item pool and direction from EC

IW participate in training and item writing workshop. IW with PTS validate, edit, and classify items according to Test Plan

PTS edits and validates items for agreement with examination specifications, psychometric properties, documentation, ethnic and sexual bias, accuracy in classification and grammar

EC selects PCE from nominees submitted by Member Boards of Nursing representing approximately ¼th of jurisdictions for RN and ¼th of jurisdictions for PN

Selection—Based on qualifications, regional distribution, and clinical practice. Boards submit nominees on a regularly scheduled basis and may participate more frequently if preferred.

PTS conducts meeting of each PCE including a representative of EC

PCE reviews appropriateness of each new item and pool items requiring updating review. Review includes documentation of content accuracy, currency, job-relatedness, appropriateness for entry-level, verification of correct answer for each item, and disposition

PTS assembles experimental items for try-out on a future examination

MB files a request to review experimental items. Review experimental items for appropriateness for entry-level practice and consistency with laws regulating nursing practice in the jurisdictions

PTS collates responses of Member Boards and conducts statistical analysis of "try-out" items

EC/PCE reviews responses from Member Boards

PTS assembles examination for administration including both "real" and "try-out" items

EC reviews examination for administration and approves for use

Key

EC—Examination Committee of the National Council of State Boards of Nursing, Inc. Members represent the areas of the National Council. One member represents a practical nursing board.

PTS—Professional Test Service under contract with the National Council.

PCE—Panel of Content Experts. Members are nominated by Member Boards and appointed by the Examination Committee. These content experts will review items to assure that understandings basic to minimum safe and effective practice are being evaluated for entry-level practical nurses.

DA—Delegate Assembly of NCSBN. Consists of representatives from each jurisdiction who govern the National Council.

IW—Item Writers. Individuals who are nominated by Member Boards and appointed by the Examination Committee.

NCSBN—National Council of State Boards of Nursing, Inc.

MB—Member Boards. Boards of Nursing in those jurisdictions which are members of the National Council of State Boards of Nursing, Inc.

NCLEX-PN

Test Plan

for the National Council

Licensure Examination

for Practical Nurses

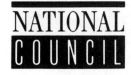

National Council
of State Boards of Nursing, Inc.

August 1989

TEST PLAN FOR THE
NATIONAL COUNCIL LICENSURE EXAMINATION FOR PRACTICAL NURSES*

Entry into the practice of nursing in the United States and its territories is regulated by the licensing authorities in the jurisdictions. Each jurisdiction requires a candidate for licensure to pass an examination that measures the competencies needed to perform safely and effectively as a newly licensed entry-level practical nurse. An entry-level practical nurse is defined as a newly licensed practical nurse who has been employed for six months or less.

Developed by the National Council of State Boards of Nursing, Inc., *The National Council Licensure Examination for Practical Nurses (NCLEX-PN)* is the examination used by those jurisdictions whose boards of nursing are National Council members.

The initial step in developing the examination for practical nurse licensure is preparation of the test plan to guide selection of content and behaviors to be tested. In the plan, provision is made for an examination reflecting entry-level nursing practice as identified by Kane and Colton in the *Job Analysis of Newly Licensed Practical/Vocational Nurses - 1986-1987.*

The activities identified in the job analysis were analyzed in relation to the frequency of their performance, their impact on maintaining client safety, the various settings in which they were performed, and the age ranges of clients.

This analysis resulted in the identification of a framework for entry-level performance that incorporates the nursing process and specific client needs and also reflects age and practice setting. The basic framework is similar to that used in the Registered Nurse Test Plan, which reflects the continuum of nursing practice. The Practical Nurse Test Plan is distinguished from the Registered Nurse Test Plan by the scope of practice as defined by member jurisdictions, by the practical nurse job analyses, and by the tested levels of cognitive abilities.

The test plan provides a concise summary of the content and scope of the examination and serves as a guide for candidates preparing to write the examination and for those individuals involved in developing it.

Based on the test plan, each assembled NCLEX-PN examination reflects the knowledge, skills, and abilities essential for application of the phases of the nursing process to meet the needs of clients with commonly occurring health problems having predictable outcomes. The following sections describe beliefs about nursing and clients, the levels of cognitive ability that will be tested in the examination, and the specific components of the NCLEX-PN test plan.

---

*The term practical nurse denotes both practical and vocational nurses.

BELIEFS

Beliefs about the nature of people and nursing underlie the test plan. Nursing has a unique concern toward helping clients to achieve an optimal state of health. Recipients of nursing care are viewed as finite beings with varying capacities to function in society. These recipients are unique persons defining their own systems of daily living that reflect values, motives, and lifestyles. Additionally, they are viewed as having the right to determine what kind of health care should be available to meet present and future needs. The consumer of nursing is an individual or group of individuals in need of assistance with maintaining life, promoting health, coping with health problems, adapting to or recovering from the effects of disease or injury, and dying with dignity.

The nature of nursing is dynamic and evolving. It is perceived as deliberate action of a personal and assisting nature. The goal of nursing is to promote health and to assist individuals in attaining an optimal level of functioning through responding to the needs, conditions, or events that result from actual or potential health problems and that provide the focus for the nurse's plan of care. The domain of nursing and the relevant knowledge, skills, and abilities exist along a continuum and are organized and defined by professional and legal parameters.

Upon entry into nursing practice, the practical nurse, under appropriate supervision, is expected to care for the client and/or assist the client's significant others in the provision of care. The practical nurse contributes to data collection for the identification of the health needs/problems of clients throughout their life cycle and in a variety of settings. Based upon established nursing diagnoses, the practical nurse contributes to planning nursing measures to meet identified needs and participates in evaluating the extent to which identified outcomes are achieved.

The practice of practical nursing requires **basic** knowledge of 1) nursing process; 2) coordination of safe, effective care; 3) client's physiological needs; 4) client's psychosocial needs; and 5) maintenance and promotion of health. The following elements are integrated throughout NCLEX-PN: accountability, nutrition, pharmacology, body structure and function, pathophysiology, principles of asepsis, growth and development, documentation, communication, teaching appropriate to the scope of practice and mental health concepts.

LEVELS OF COGNITIVE ABILITY

The examination includes test items at the cognitive levels of knowledge, comprehension, and application. Weighing (i.e., the number of items assigned to each level) is not specified for the levels of cognitive ability; however, most items in the examination are at the comprehension and application levels.

COMPONENTS OF THE TEST PLAN

Two components are addressed within the framework of the test plan: 1) phase of the nursing process; and 2) client needs. These are described in the following sections.

PHASES OF THE NURSING PROCESS

The phases of the nursing process are grouped under the broad categories of collecting data, planning, implementing, and evaluating nursing care. The practical nurse assists with the collection of data about the client, contributes to the client's plan of care, performs basic therapeutic and preventive nursing measures, and assists in evaluating the outcomes of nursing interventions.

The entry-level practical nurse acts in a more dependent role when participating in the planning and evaluation phases of the nursing process and acts in a more independent role when participating in the data collecting and implementing phases of the nursing process. Therefore, the percentages of questions representing the various phases of the nursing process are as follows: 1) collecting data - 30%; 2) planning - 20%; 3) implementing - 30%; 4) evaluating - 20%.

I.   In collecting data about clients with commonly occurring health problems having predictable outcomes, the practical nurse:

    A.   Contributes to the development of a data base about clients by:

        1.   Observing the physiological, psychosocial, health and safety needs of clients.

        2.   Collecting information from the client, significant others, health team members and records.

        3.   Determining the need for more information.

        4.   Communicating findings of data collected.

    B.   Participates in the formulation of nursing diagnoses.

II.   In planning care for clients with commonly occurring health problems having predictable outcomes, the practical nurse:

    A.   Contributes to the development of nursing care plans for clients with health needs.

B. Assists in the formulation of goals.

C. Participates in the identification of clients' needs and nursing measures required to achieve goals.

D. Communicates needs that may require alteration of the care plan.

E. Communicates with the client, significant others and/or health team members in planning nursing care.

III. In implementing care for clients with commonly occurring health problems having predictable outcomes, the practical nurse:

A. Performs basic therapeutic and preventive nursing measures by following a prescribed plan of care to achieve established client goals.

B. Provides a safe and effective environment.

C. Assists client, significant others and health care members to understand the client's plan of care.

D. Records client information and reports it to other health team members.

IV. In evaluating care of clients with commonly occurring health problems having predictable outcomes, the practical nurse:

A. Participates in evaluating the effectiveness of the client's nursing care.

B. Assists in evaluating the client's response to nursing care and in making appropriate alterations.

C. Evaluates the extent to which identified outcomes of the care plan are achieved.

D. Records and describes client's responses to therapy and/or care.

CLIENT NEEDS

The health needs of clients are grouped under four broad categories: A) safe, effective care environment; B) physiological integrity; C) psychosocial integrity; and D) health promotion/maintenance. The weighing of these categories was based on an analysis of the results of a job analysis study completed in 1987. Thus, the percentage of items assigned to each category of client need is as follows:

A.	Safe, effective care environment	24-30 percent
B.	Physiological integrity	42-48 percent
C.	Psychosocial integrity	7-13 percent
D.	Health promotion and maintenance	15-21 percent

A. Safe, Effective Care Environment

The practical nurse participates as a member of the health care team to assist in meeting client needs for a safe and effective environment by providing nursing care to clients with common health problems that occur throughout the life cycle and have predictable outcomes in the following categories:

1. Coordinated care

2. Standards of care

3. Goal-oriented care

4. Environmental safety

5. Preparation for treatments and procedures

6. Safe and effective treatments and procedures

Knowledge, Skills, and Abilities

In order to meet client needs for a safe and effective environment, the practical nurse should possess **basic** knowledge, skills, and abilities that include but are not limited to the following examples:

knowledge of data-gathering techniques; interpersonal communication skills; alternative methods of communication for clients with special needs; client preparation for prescribed treatments and procedures; environmental and client safety; infection control; client rights; confidentiality; individualization of care, including religious, cultural, and developmental influences; team participation in care planning and evaluation and general knowledge of community agencies.

B. **Physiological Integrity**
The practical nurse participates as a member of the health care team to assist in meeting the physiological needs of clients with common health problems that occur throughout the life cycle and have predictable outcomes. This includes clients with acute and chronic conditions and clients at risk for the development of complications. Nursing care is provided to promote achievement of the following client needs:

7. Physiological adaptation

8. Reduction of risk potential

9. Mobility

10. Comfort

11. Provisions of basic care

Knowledge, Skills, and Abilities
In order to meet client needs for physiological integrity, the practical nurse should possess **basic** knowledge, skills, and abilities in areas that include but are not limited to the following examples:

knowledge of therapeutic and life-saving procedures, specialized equipment, principles of administering medications, maintenance of optimal body functioning and prevention of complications, principles of body mechanics and assistive devices, comfort measures, routine nursing measures and reporting changes in a client's condition.

C. **Psychosocial Integrity**
The practical nurse participates as a member of the health care team to assist in meeting the psychosocial needs of clients with common health problems that occur throughout the life cycle and have predictable outcomes. Nursing care is provided to promote achievement of the following client needs:

12. Psychosocial adaptation

13. Coping/Adaptation

Knowledge, Skills, and Abilities
In order to meet client needs for psychosocial integrity, the practical nurse should possess **basic** knowledge, skills, and abilities in areas that include but are not limited to the following examples:

> obvious signs of emotional and mental health problems, self-concept, life crises, chemical dependency, adaptive and maladaptive behavior, sensory deprivation and overload, abusive and self-destructive behavior, therapeutic communication, common therapies and general knowledge of community resources.

D.   Health Promotion/Maintenance
The practical nurse participates as a member of the health care team to assist in meeting health promotion and maintenance needs of clients with common health problems that occur throughout the life cycle and have predictable outcomes. Nursing care is provided to promote fulfillment of the following client needs:

14.   Continued growth and development

15.   Self-care

16.   Integrity of support system

17.   Prevention and early treatment of disease

Knowledge, Skills, and Abilities
In order to meet client needs for health promotion/maintenance, the practical nurse should possess **basic** knowledge, skills, and abilities in areas that include but are not limited to the following:

> family interactions; concepts of wellness; adaptation to altered health states; reproduction and human sexuality; birthing and parenting; growth and development, including dying and death; immunization; health teaching that is appropriate to the scope of practice; and general knowledge of community resources.

REFERENCES

Bloom, B.S., et al. (1956). _Taxonomy of Educational Objectives: The Classification of Educational Goals, Handbook._ 1. New York: David McKay.

Competencies of Graduates of Educational Programs in Practical Nursing. (1979). New York: National League for Nursing.

Hood, G. and Dincher, J. (1984). _Total Patient Care: Foundations and Practice._ St. Louis: C.V. Mosby.

"Hypothesized Entry-Level Competency Statements for Evolving Levels of Nursing Practice." _Delegate Assembly Book of Reports._ (1988). Chicago: National Council of State Boards of Nursing, Inc. pp. 207-213.

Kane, M., Kingsbury, C., Colton, D., and Estes, C. (1986). _A Study of Nursing Practice and Role Delineation, and Job Analysis of Entry-Level Performance of Registered Nurses._ Chicago: National Council of State Boards of Nursing, Inc.

Kane, M. and Colton, D. (1988). _Job Analysis of Newly Licensed Practical/Vocational Nurses, 1986-87._ Chicago: National Council of State Boards of Nursing, Inc.

Keane, C. (1986). _Essentials of Medical-Surgical Nursing._ Philadelphia: W.B. Saunders.

Rosedahl, C. (1985). _Textbook of Basic Nursing._ New York: J.B. Lippincott.

Scherer, J. (1986). _Introductory Medical-Surgical Nursing._ New York: J.B. Lippincott.